MW00954566

THE LOST CASTOR OIL BIBLE

Unlocking all the Secrets of the Most Effective Ancient Natural Elixir |+100 Castor Oil Recipes and Remedies to Achieve Your Health, Wellness and Beauty Goals.

Eliza Green

GET YOUR BONUS NOW!

BONUS:

NATURAL CREATIONS: DIY BATH, BODY, and HERBAL ESSENTIALS - Ebook

Go to page 132...

SCAN the QR code and

DOWNLOAD your amazing

BONUS

Table of Contents

Chapter 1: Introduction to Castor Oil

Castor oil, derived from the seeds of the Ricinus communis plant, has been revered for centuries across various cultures for its remarkable healing properties. This natural elixir, with its rich history dating back to ancient Egypt, was traditionally used for its anti-inflammatory and antibacterial benefits, making it a staple in traditional medicine cabinets. The versatility of castor oil extends beyond medicinal uses; it's also celebrated for its beauty-enhancing properties, providing a natural solution for skin and hair care enthusiasts seeking to avoid harsh chemicals.

Understanding the basics of castor oil involves recognizing the different types available on the market—cold-pressed, organic, and hexane-free, each with its own set of benefits. Cold-pressed castor oil, obtained by pressing the seeds without heat, retains most of its nutritional content, making it highly sought after for therapeutic uses. Organic castor oil ensures that the seeds were grown without the use of pesticides or chemical fertilizers, offering a pure, toxin-free product. Hexane-free castor oil indicates that the extraction process did not involve hexane, a solvent that can leave behind harmful residues.

The extraction methods of castor oil play a crucial role in determining its quality and efficacy. Cold-pressing is the most traditional and effective method, preserving the oil's natural healing properties. This method ensures that the oil maintains its high levels of ricinoleic acid, the key component responsible for its anti-inflammatory and pain-relieving effects. Understanding these basics provides a solid foundation for exploring the vast therapeutic applications and incorporating castor oil into daily health and beauty routines, promising a holistic approach to wellness that harnesses the power of nature's most effective ancient elixir.

The Origins and History of Castor Oil

Tracing the origins of castor oil leads us back to ancient civilizations where it was not just a medicinal elixir but a symbol of healing and protection. Extracted from the seeds of the Ricinus communis plant, castor oil's journey began in the warm regions of Africa and India, where it was first cultivated and used. Ancient Egyptian tombs, including that of Tutankhamun, have revealed papyrus scrolls dating back to 1550 B.C., which document the use of castor oil for lighting lamps and as an ointment to protect the eyes from irritation. Its versatility was recognized early on, with uses ranging from an ingredient in skin ointments to an agent for inducing labor.

The castor plant, known as "Palma Christe" because the leaves were thought to resemble the hand of Christ, was revered for its healing powers. In India, it has been a staple in Ayurvedic medicine for thousands of years, utilized for its anti-inflammatory and antibacterial properties. The healing traditions of Greece and Rome also embraced castor oil, employing it as a wound healer and laxative.

By the turn of the 19th century, castor oil found its way into the American pharmacopeia, becoming a household remedy for various ailments, particularly as a natural laxative. Its role in industry expanded during the World Wars, when it was used as a lubricant for aircraft engines.

Today, castor oil continues to be a valued component in the pharmaceutical, cosmetic, and manufacturing industries, thanks to its unique chemical composition. The journey of castor oil, from an ancient remedy to a modern-day marvel, underscores its enduring legacy as one of nature's most versatile and effective elixirs. Its history is a testament to the timeless search for natural solutions to health and beauty, a search that continues to inspire and guide us.

Basics of Types and Extraction

When delving into the world of castor oil, it's essential to understand the different types available and the methods used to extract this potent oil. Each type of castor oil has unique characteristics and benefits, making it suitable for various applications, from health and beauty remedies to therapeutic uses. The extraction method also plays a crucial role in determining the quality and efficacy of the oil, influencing its chemical composition and, consequently, its healing properties.

Cold-pressed castor oil is the most common and widely appreciated for its purity and nutritional content. This method involves pressing the seeds of the Ricinus communis plant without the use of heat, thereby preserving the essential nutrients and enzymes. Cold-pressed castor oil is rich in ricinoleic acid, a unique fatty acid that contributes to its anti-inflammatory and antibacterial properties. It's ideal for medicinal and skincare applications, offering a natural, potent remedy for a range of conditions.

Organic castor oil takes the benefits of cold-pressing a step further by ensuring that the castor seeds are grown without the use of synthetic pesticides or fertilizers. This not only makes the oil safer for use but also supports sustainable farming practices. Organic castor oil is preferred by those looking to maintain an eco-friendly lifestyle while enjoying the therapeutic benefits of castor oil.

Hexane-free castor oil addresses concerns about solvent residues in the oil. Hexane, a chemical solvent, is sometimes used in the extraction process to increase oil yield. However, traces of hexane can remain in the oil, posing potential health risks. Hexane-free castor oil guarantees that no chemical solvents were used during extraction, offering a cleaner, safer product.

The extraction method significantly impacts the oil's quality. Cold-pressing is the most effective method to retain the therapeutic properties of castor oil. In contrast, solvent extraction methods, such as using hexane, can degrade the oil's quality and reduce its beneficial properties.

Understanding these basics is crucial for anyone looking to incorporate castor oil into their health and beauty routines. Whether you're seeking a natural remedy for skin conditions, looking to enhance hair health, or exploring its therapeutic benefits, choosing the right type of castor oil and understanding its extraction method can make a significant difference in achieving your wellness goals. With this knowledge, you can confidently navigate the vast array of castor oil products available, ensuring you select the best option for your specific needs.

Chapter 2: The Science Behind Castor Oil

Delving into the science behind castor oil reveals why it has been such a revered natural remedy throughout history. The key to its therapeutic prowess lies in its unique chemical composition, primarily consisting of ricinoleic acid, a rare and highly beneficial fatty acid. Ricinoleic acid accounts for about 90% of castor oil's fatty acid content, setting it apart from other plant oils. Its structure allows it to penetrate deep into the skin, providing hydration and helping to maintain skin health by promoting the growth of healthy tissue. This fatty acid is also responsible for castor oil's anti-inflammatory properties, making it an effective treatment for conditions like arthritis, inflammatory bowel syndrome, and dermatitis.

Beyond ricinoleic acid, castor oil contains other important components such as oleic, linoleic, stearic, and palmitic acids, though in much smaller quantities. These fatty acids contribute to the oil's overall health benefits, including moisturizing effects, support for hair growth, and the reduction of inflammation. Additionally, castor oil is rich in antioxidants, which combat free radicals in the body, reducing oxidative stress and lowering the risk of chronic diseases.

The therapeutic uses and applications of castor oil are vast and varied. Its anti-inflammatory and antibacterial properties make it an excellent remedy for acne, as it can reduce swelling, redness, and bacteria associated with breakouts. Castor oil is also known for its ability to stimulate the lymphatic system, enhancing the body's detoxification processes. This stimulation is particularly beneficial for the immune system, as it helps to produce more lymphocytes, the body's natural disease-fighters.

For digestive health, castor oil acts as a stimulant laxative, providing relief from constipation by increasing the movement of the muscles that push material through the intestines. However, it's important to use it correctly, as excessive use can lead to electrolyte imbalance and loss of muscle function in the intestines.

In terms of pain relief, castor oil's anti-inflammatory properties make it an effective natural treatment for joint pain, nerve inflammation, and sore muscles. Applying it topically in the form of a castor oil pack can significantly reduce pain and inflammation without the side effects associated with over-the-counter pain medications.

The science behind castor oil also extends to its use in hair and scalp treatments. Its ability to moisturize and promote circulation to the scalp can lead to healthier hair growth, while its antifungal properties help to combat dandruff and other scalp conditions.

Understanding the scientific foundation of castor oil's benefits allows for a deeper appreciation of its potential as a natural remedy. Its unique chemical makeup and the body's response to these components underscore the importance of incorporating castor oil into a holistic approach to health and wellness. With a clear grasp of the science behind castor oil, individuals can make informed decisions about how to effectively use this ancient elixir to enhance their health and beauty routines, harnessing its natural power to address a wide range of conditions.

Chemical Composition and Properties

The chemical composition of castor oil is a fascinating blend of components, each contributing to its remarkable therapeutic properties. At the heart of castor oil's effectiveness is ricinoleic acid, a monounsaturated fatty acid that comprises about 90% of the oil's fatty acid content. This unique fatty acid is what sets castor oil apart from other plant oils and is the key to its powerful health benefits.

In addition to ricinoleic acid, castor oil contains smaller amounts of other fatty acids including oleic, linoleic, stearic, and palmitic acids. Oleic acid contributes to the oil's moisturizing and regenerative capabilities, while linoleic acid offers anti-inflammatory benefits and helps maintain healthy skin. Stearic and palmitic acids play a role in softening the skin and stabilizing the oil's consistency, enhancing its applicability in cosmetic formulations.

The antioxidant content in castor oil further amplifies its health benefits. Antioxidants combat oxidative stress in the body by neutralizing free radicals, molecules that can damage cells and contribute to aging and diseases. By reducing oxidative stress, castor oil supports overall health and helps protect the skin and hair from environmental damage.

Castor oil's molecular weight and structure allow it to penetrate deeply into the skin and scalp, delivering its therapeutic compounds directly to the cells that need them most. This ability to penetrate beyond the surface makes castor oil an effective moisturizer and healing agent, capable of reaching underlying tissues to soothe inflammation, hydrate skin cells, and promote healing.

The viscosity of castor oil, which is relatively high compared to other plant oils, is another important aspect of its composition. This thickness is beneficial when the oil is used in hair and scalp treatments, as it coats the hair thoroughly and provides a protective barrier against moisture loss. The viscosity also makes castor oil an excellent carrier oil for blending with essential oils, enhancing the effectiveness of both the castor oil and the essential oils.

Understanding the chemical composition and properties of castor oil provides valuable insights into its health benefits and therapeutic applications. By appreciating the science behind this ancient natural remedy, individuals can make informed decisions about incorporating castor oil into their wellness and beauty routines. Whether used for its anti-inflammatory effects, its ability to moisturize and regenerate skin and hair, or its protective antioxidant properties, castor oil offers a natural, effective solution for a wide range of health and beauty concerns.

Chapter 3: Castor Oil Packs

Castor oil packs, a traditional remedy passed down through generations, have been celebrated for their ability to enhance health and wellness significantly. These packs leverage the potent anti-inflammatory and lymphatic-stimulating properties of castor oil, offering a simple yet effective method for addressing a variety of health concerns. The application of a castor oil pack can provide relief from pain, reduce inflammation, support digestive health, and promote detoxification of the body. This chapter delves into the practical aspects of creating and using castor oil packs, providing readers with a comprehensive guide to harnessing the therapeutic benefits of castor oil in a safe and effective manner.

Objective: To educate on the preparation, application, and benefits of castor oil packs, enabling individuals to incorporate this natural remedy into their health and wellness routines.

Preparation:
1. Select high-quality, cold-pressed, organic castor oil to ensure maximum purity and effectiveness.
2. Choose a piece of soft, natural fabric such as wool or cotton flannel large enough to cover the targeted area.
3. Have a plastic wrap or a plastic bag cut to size to cover the cloth soaked in castor oil.
4. Prepare a hot water bottle or heating pad to apply warmth over the pack.
5. Ensure the area of application on the body is clean and free of any products.

Materials:
- Cold-pressed, organic castor oil
- Wool or cotton flannel
- Plastic wrap or plastic bag
- Hot water bottle or heating pad
- Old clothes and sheets (castor oil can stain)

Tools:
- Glass bowl or container for soaking the cloth in castor oil
- Measuring cup for castor oil
- Scissors (if fabric needs to be cut to size)

Safety measures:
- Conduct a patch test to rule out any allergic reactions to castor oil.
- Avoid using castor oil packs during pregnancy and menstruation.
- Do not apply castor oil packs to broken skin or open wounds.
- Ensure the heating element is not too hot to prevent burns.

Step-by-step instructions:
1. Pour an adequate amount of castor oil into the glass bowl. The quantity depends on the size of the flannel and the area of application.

2. Soak the flannel in castor oil until it is fully saturated but not dripping.
3. Place the soaked flannel over the targeted area, such as the abdomen for digestive issues or the joints for pain relief.
4. Cover the flannel with plastic wrap to prevent staining and to hold the pack in place.
5. Place the hot water bottle or heating pad over the plastic wrap to apply gentle heat.
6. Leave the castor oil pack on for 45-60 minutes, relaxing during this time to enhance the therapeutic effects.
7. Remove the pack and cleanse the area with a warm, damp towel. Washing with a solution of baking soda and water can help remove oil residues.
8. Store the used flannel in a plastic bag in the refrigerator. The flannel can be reused multiple times, adding more oil as needed.

Cost estimate: The initial setup cost is minimal, primarily involving the purchase of castor oil and a piece of flannel. These materials, along with the heating element, can be used multiple times, making castor oil packs a cost-effective remedy.

Time estimate: Preparation time is about 5-10 minutes, with each session lasting 45-60 minutes. Including cleanup, the total time commitment per session is approximately 1-1.5 hours.

Safety tips:
- Always test the temperature of the heating pad or hot water bottle before application.
- Start with shorter sessions to assess tolerance before increasing to longer durations.
- Consult with a healthcare provider before using castor oil packs for specific health conditions.

Troubleshooting:
- If irritation occurs, reduce the duration of application or discontinue use.
- Should castor oil stain fabrics or furniture, applying baking soda and dish soap before laundering can help remove stains.

Maintenance: Rinse and air dry the flannel after each use, storing it in a cool, dry place. Regularly check the heating element for any signs of wear or damage.

Difficulty rating: ★☆☆☆☆

Variations: For enhanced therapeutic effects, essential oils such as lavender or peppermint can be added to the castor oil. Adjust the size of the flannel and the amount of castor oil based on the specific area being treated.

By following these guidelines, individuals can effectively utilize castor oil packs as a natural remedy to support their health and wellness. This traditional practice, rooted in centuries of holistic healing, offers a gentle yet powerful approach to addressing a wide range of health concerns, embodying the essence of natural, self-directed healthcare.

The Role of Castor Oil Packs

Castor oil packs have long been a cornerstone in the world of natural healing, praised for their ability to draw out toxins, ease pain, and stimulate lymphatic circulation. Their role in holistic health practices is rooted in the understanding that the body can heal itself when given the right support. Castor oil, with its unique composition, particularly the high content of ricinoleic acid, serves as a powerful tool in this self-healing process. When applied as a pack, castor oil works deeply, not just on the physical level to relieve pain or inflammation, but also on a subtle level, aiding in the detoxification and rejuvenation of tissues. This dual action makes castor oil packs an invaluable addition to anyone's wellness regimen, particularly for those dealing with chronic conditions or seeking to enhance their body's natural detoxification processes.

The effectiveness of castor oil packs lies in their ability to penetrate the skin and improve the body's absorption of the oil's therapeutic properties. The warmth applied over the pack helps in opening the pores of the skin, ensuring that the ricinoleic acid and other beneficial components of castor oil are absorbed more efficiently. This process can significantly enhance circulation in the lymphatic system, a critical part of the body's immune system. By improving lymphatic flow, castor oil packs contribute to reducing swelling, enhancing organ function, and promoting the removal of toxins from the body. This mechanism of action is particularly beneficial for improving digestive health, as the packs are often applied to the abdomen to stimulate liver function, relieve constipation, and reduce bloating.

Moreover, the anti-inflammatory properties of castor oil make these packs an excellent choice for pain management. Whether it's joint pain, menstrual cramps, or headaches, the application of a castor oil pack can provide natural and effective relief. The oil's ability to soothe inflammation and reduce pain is complemented by its potential to enhance the healing of tissues, making it a versatile remedy for a wide range of conditions.

While castor oil packs are generally safe for most people, it's important to be mindful of potential allergies and to avoid their use in certain conditions, such as during pregnancy or over broken skin. As with any natural remedy, listening to one's body and consulting with a healthcare provider if necessary is crucial to ensure safety and effectiveness.

The role of castor oil packs extends beyond their physical benefits, touching on the emotional and mental aspects of health as well. The act of taking time to care for oneself, to relax and to focus on healing, can have profound effects on one's mental state and emotional well-being. In this way, castor oil packs not only offer a method for addressing specific health issues but also serve as a practice of holistic self-care, embodying the principles of natural healing and the body's innate capacity for regeneration.

Chapter 4: Castor Oil Health Benefits

Harnessing the power of castor oil for health benefits is akin to unlocking an ancient treasure trove of natural remedies that have stood the test of time.

Immune system support is one of the most celebrated benefits of castor oil. Its ability to increase the production of lymphocytes, white blood cells that play a critical role in the body's defense mechanisms, is particularly noteworthy. This boost in lymphocyte count not only strengthens the immune system but also helps in detoxifying the body, making castor oil a powerful ally in maintaining overall health and warding off diseases.

The versatility of castor oil extends to a range of applications, from turmeric pain relief balms to ginger compresses, each designed to harness the oil's natural properties for specific health benefits. Whether it's a eucalyptus massage oil for muscle relaxation, a peppermint foot soak for revitalization, or a lavender relaxation bath to soothe the senses, castor oil's adaptability makes it a cornerstone ingredient in natural health and wellness practices.

As we delve deeper into the myriad health benefits of castor oil, it's clear that its potential goes beyond mere topical applications. Its role in enhancing overall wellness, supporting the immune system, and providing natural solutions for pain and inflammation showcases the timeless relevance of this ancient remedy. With each use, castor oil continues to reveal its profound capabilities, making it a staple in the pursuit of natural health and beauty.

Building on the foundation of castor oil's remarkable benefits for immune support, digestive health, and pain relief, its role in promoting respiratory health emerges as another key aspect of its therapeutic versatility. Castor oil's anti-inflammatory properties can be particularly beneficial for those suffering from respiratory conditions such as asthma or bronchitis. By applying a castor oil pack to the chest, individuals may experience eased breathing and reduced inflammation in the airways, offering a gentle, natural method to support respiratory wellness.

The benefits of castor oil extend into the realm of mental health as well. Its use in aromatherapy, often as a carrier oil blended with essential oils like lavender or peppermint, can have a calming effect on the mind, reducing stress and anxiety. This soothing property not only enhances mental well-being but also supports sleep quality. Incorporating castor oil into nighttime routines, perhaps through a massage or a warm bath, can help ease the transition into restful sleep, addressing issues of insomnia and promoting overall relaxation.

For women's health, castor oil offers specific advantages, particularly in the management of menstrual discomfort and in supporting reproductive health. Applying a castor oil pack to the lower abdomen can help alleviate menstrual cramps and reduce inflammation, offering a comforting remedy during periods of discomfort. Additionally, its circulatory benefits can support reproductive health by promoting blood flow to the reproductive organs, which is beneficial for women experiencing irregular menstrual cycles or those seeking to enhance fertility naturally.

Finally, the detoxifying properties of castor oil should not be overlooked. Its ability to stimulate the lymphatic system aids in the removal of toxins from the body, supporting liver function and enhancing the body's natural detoxification processes. This, in turn, can have a positive impact on overall health and vitality, reflecting in clearer skin, improved energy levels, and a strengthened immune system.

Through its wide-ranging applications and health benefits, castor oil stands out as a versatile and powerful natural remedy. Its ability to address a broad spectrum of health concerns, from physical ailments to mental wellness, underscores the enduring value of this ancient elixir. Embracing castor oil in daily wellness practices can unlock a path to natural, holistic health, reflecting the timeless wisdom encapsulated in this remarkable oil.

Immune System Support

Boosting the immune system is a critical aspect of maintaining overall health and wellness, and castor oil, with its unique composition, plays a significant role in enhancing the body's natural defense mechanisms. Rich in ricinoleic acid, castor oil has been shown to stimulate the production of lymphocytes, which are pivotal in the body's fight against infections and diseases. Lymphocytes, part of the white blood cells, are essential for producing antibodies that combat pathogens, making castor oil a potent ally in strengthening the immune system.

The application of castor oil packs, a traditional and effective method, directly supports lymphatic drainage and immune function. By applying a castor oil pack to the abdomen, you can help increase lymphatic circulation, which in turn aids in the removal of toxins from the body. This detoxification process is crucial for a healthy immune system as it helps to reduce the body's toxic burden and supports the function of the liver, a key organ in the body's defense system.

Moreover, the anti-inflammatory properties of castor oil contribute to its immune-supporting capabilities. Inflammation is a natural response of the body's immune system to injury or infection, but chronic inflammation can lead to a host of health issues and weaken the immune system. By applying castor oil topically, you can help reduce inflammation, providing a healthier environment for the immune system to function effectively.

Digestive System Health

Castor oil offers a natural and effective remedy for a variety of digestive issues, making it a valuable addition to anyone's wellness toolkit. Its ability to act as a stimulant laxative is perhaps the most well-known benefit, providing relief from constipation and helping to maintain regular bowel movements. However, its benefits for digestive health extend far beyond this single application. The anti-inflammatory properties of castor oil can soothe irritated intestines, reducing discomfort from bloating and gas, while its antimicrobial effects help in balancing the gut flora, essential for a healthy digestive system.

For individuals dealing with constipation, incorporating castor oil into their routine can offer significant relief. The mechanism behind its laxative effect involves the ricinoleic acid binding to the smooth muscle cells of the intestinal walls, stimulating a strong laxative effect that promotes the movement of stool through the intestines. This can alleviate the discomfort associated with constipation and help restore regular bowel movements.

To utilize castor oil for constipation relief, a simple method involves taking a small amount of cold-pressed, organic castor oil orally. It's important to start with a low dose, as the potency of castor oil can vary greatly among individuals. A typical starting point might be one teaspoon, taken on an empty stomach, to assess tolerance. For some, increasing the dose slightly may be necessary, but it's crucial to not exceed the recommended dosage as outlined by a healthcare professional to avoid adverse effects.

Materials needed for this application include:
- Cold-pressed, organic castor oil
- Measuring spoon

Safety measures are paramount when ingesting castor oil. It should not be used as a long-term solution for constipation without consulting a healthcare provider. Pregnant women, breastfeeding mothers, and individuals with intestinal blockages or acute inflammatory intestinal diseases should avoid ingesting castor oil due to potential risks.

For those interested in topical application to support digestive health, castor oil packs are a gentle and effective method. This method can help in enhancing circulation, reducing inflammation, and promoting healing in the digestive tract.

Using castor oil, whether orally or through packs, can support digestive health by improving bowel movements, reducing inflammation, and aiding in the maintenance of a balanced gut microbiome. However, it's essential to approach its use with caution, adhering to recommended dosages and consulting a healthcare provider, especially in cases of severe or chronic digestive issues. Through mindful use, castor oil can be a powerful tool in achieving and maintaining optimal digestive health, contributing to overall well-being.

Pain Relief and Anti-Inflammatory Effects

Understanding Pain and Inflammation

Pain and inflammation are two of the most common health complaints that affect millions of people worldwide. They can result from various conditions, including arthritis, muscle strains, menstrual cramps, and chronic diseases. While modern medicine offers numerous solutions for pain and inflammation, many of these come with significant side effects and long-term health risks. This is where castor oil, a natural remedy used for centuries, comes into play. Known for its potent anti-inflammatory and analgesic properties, castor oil can provide a natural alternative for managing pain and reducing inflammation.

- **Anti-inflammatory Effects**: Ricinoleic acid inhibits the production of pro-inflammatory markers in the body, such as prostaglandins, which play a key role in the inflammation process. By reducing the levels of these markers, castor oil helps to diminish inflammation and its associated symptoms.

- **Analgesic Properties**: Apart from its anti-inflammatory effects, ricinoleic acid also acts as an analgesic, helping to relieve pain. It interacts with sensory neurons and reduces the sensation of pain by blocking the transmission of pain signals to the brain.
- **Antioxidant Activity**: Castor oil is also rich in antioxidants, which help to neutralize free radicals and reduce oxidative stress in the body. This is particularly beneficial in preventing and managing chronic inflammatory conditions.

Alleviating Arthritis Pain

Arthritis is a common condition characterized by joint pain and inflammation. Castor oil is particularly effective in managing arthritis pain due to its high ricinoleic acid content, which possesses powerful anti-inflammatory properties. Regular application of castor oil to the affected joints can help reduce swelling and alleviate pain. The oil penetrates deep into the tissues, improving blood circulation and reducing stiffness.

To use castor oil for arthritis, gently massage it into the painful joints. For enhanced benefits, you can wrap the area with a warm cloth or castor oil pack, allowing the oil to penetrate deeply and provide prolonged relief. This method not only soothes pain but also helps to improve joint flexibility over time.

Relieving Muscle Strain and Soreness

Muscle strain and soreness can occur from overexertion, exercise, or injury. Castor oil can be a valuable ally in soothing these aches. Its natural anti-inflammatory and analgesic properties make it an excellent choice for relieving muscle pain.

To address muscle soreness, warm a small amount of castor oil and massage it into the affected muscles. The warmth helps the oil to absorb better, providing deeper relief. This practice can be particularly beneficial after a workout or a long day of physical activity, helping to speed up recovery and reduce discomfort.

Easing Menstrual Cramps

Menstrual cramps are a common issue for many women, often causing significant discomfort. Castor oil can help ease these cramps by reducing inflammation and relaxing the muscles. Applying a warm castor oil pack to the lower abdomen can provide soothing relief.

To use castor oil for menstrual cramps, soak a cloth in warm castor oil, place it on the lower abdomen, cover it with plastic wrap, and apply a heating pad or hot water bottle. Leave the pack on for about an hour. This method helps to reduce pain and can be used regularly during the menstrual cycle to manage discomfort effectively.

Treating Chronic Pain Conditions

Chronic pain conditions, such as fibromyalgia and lower back pain, can significantly impact quality of life. Castor oil's anti-inflammatory and pain-relieving properties offer a natural way to manage chronic pain without relying on pharmaceuticals.

For chronic pain relief, apply castor oil to the affected area daily. Over time, the oil can help to reduce inflammation and pain, promoting better mobility and a higher quality of life. Regular use can also help to prevent flare-ups and maintain a more consistent level of comfort.

Anti-Inflammatory Benefits

Inflammation is a natural response to injury or infection, but chronic inflammation can lead to various health issues, including pain. Castor oil is effective in reducing chronic inflammation, making it a valuable addition to any pain management regimen.

The anti-inflammatory effects of castor oil are due to its ability to inhibit the production of pro-inflammatory compounds in the body. Regular use can help to manage conditions like rheumatoid arthritis, where inflammation is a primary concern. Applying castor oil to inflamed areas can provide significant relief, reducing redness, swelling, and pain.

Enhancing Recovery from Injuries

Injuries, whether from sports, accidents, or daily activities, often result in pain and inflammation. Castor oil can aid in the recovery process by reducing inflammation and promoting healing. Its properties help to increase blood flow to the injured area, speeding up the healing process and reducing recovery time.

To use castor oil for injury recovery, apply it to the injured area and cover with a warm cloth. The heat helps the oil to penetrate deeply, providing more effective relief and promoting faster healing.

By understanding how to use castor oil properly, you can take advantage of its potent properties to improve your quality of life and find relief from persistent pain and inflammation.

Additional Health Benefits

Expanding beyond its well-documented roles in immune support, digestive health, and pain relief, castor oil's spectrum of health benefits stretches into areas that might surprise even the most health-conscious individuals. Its utility in enhancing circulatory health, supporting the endocrine system, aiding in skin conditions beyond the common acne and dryness, and even its potential in mental health and wellness, underscores the versatility and power of this ancient remedy.

Castor oil's positive impact on circulatory health is rooted in its ability to promote blood flow, which is essential for the nourishment and oxygenation of tissues throughout the body. Improved circulation not only aids in the healing of tissues and reduction of inflammation but also supports heart health and the detoxification processes. For those seeking to enhance their circulatory health, incorporating castor oil into their routine through topical application or castor oil packs can be a simple yet effective strategy.

The endocrine system, which is pivotal in regulating hormones, can also benefit from the regular use of castor oil. Its application, particularly in the form of packs, is believed to stimulate the lymphatic and circulatory systems, which in turn can help in balancing hormone levels. This is particularly relevant for thyroid health, where castor oil packs applied to the neck may support thyroid function and, by extension, overall metabolic health.

Skin conditions such as eczema and psoriasis, can also find relief through the antimicrobial and anti-inflammatory properties of castor oil. Regular application of castor oil to affected areas can help to soothe irritation, reduce redness and swelling, and promote the healing of the skin.

Mental health and wellness, while not typically associated with the application of oils, can benefit from the use of castor oil due to its soothing properties. When used in aromatherapy or as part of a relaxing massage, castor oil can help to alleviate stress and anxiety, promote relaxation, and improve sleep quality. This calming effect is not only beneficial for mental health but can also contribute to physical health by reducing stress-induced inflammation and supporting immune function.

For individuals interested in exploring the additional health benefits of castor oil, here are practical ways to incorporate it into your health and wellness routine:

1. **Circulatory Health**: Apply castor oil directly to the skin, massaging in a circular motion towards the heart to promote blood circulation. For enhanced effects, use warm castor oil or cover the applied area with a warm cloth.
2. **Endocrine System Support**: Use castor oil packs over the abdomen to support detoxification and hormone balance. Soak a cloth in castor oil, apply it to the lower abdomen, cover with plastic wrap, and place a heating pad or hot water bottle on top for 45-60 minutes.
3. **Skin Conditions**: Apply castor oil directly to affected areas of the skin to soothe irritation, moisturize, and reduce inflammation. For conditions like fungal infections, consider blending castor oil with antifungal essential oils like tea tree oil for added benefits.
4. **Mental Wellness**: Incorporate castor oil into a relaxing massage routine or add it to bathwater for a soothing and stress-relieving experience. Blending castor oil with calming essential oils like lavender can enhance its stress-reducing effects.

By exploring these additional health benefits, individuals can unlock new dimensions of wellness with castor oil, leveraging its ancient healing properties to address a wide range of modern health concerns.

Chapter 5: Natural Castor Oil Recipes for Health and Beauty

Skin Health and Beauty Recipes

Castor Oil and Rosehip Seed Oil Brightening Serum

Beneficial effects

The Castor Oil and Rosehip Seed Oil Brightening Serum is a potent blend designed to enhance skin radiance, reduce dark spots, and improve overall skin tone. Castor oil, known for its skin-healing properties, deeply moisturizes and helps to fade blemishes, while rosehip seed oil, rich in vitamins A and C, promotes cell regeneration and boosts skin luminosity. Together, they create a powerful serum that not only brightens the skin but also provides anti-aging benefits, improving texture and reducing the appearance of fine lines and wrinkles.

Ingredients
- 2 tablespoons of cold-pressed castor oil
- 2 tablespoons of cold-pressed rosehip seed oil
- 5 drops of lemon essential oil (optional for added brightening and clarifying properties)
- 2 drops of lavender essential oil (optional for soothing and anti-inflammatory effects)
- Dark glass dropper bottle

Instructions
1. In a small bowl, thoroughly mix the castor oil and rosehip seed oil.
2. If using, add the lemon and lavender essential oils to the oil blend. These essential oils can enhance the brightening effects and add a calming, pleasant scent to the serum.
3. Carefully pour the mixture into the dark glass dropper bottle to protect the oils from light degradation.
4. To use, apply 2-3 drops of the serum to clean, damp skin at night, gently massaging in upward motions until fully absorbed. Avoid direct sunlight after applying, especially if using lemon essential oil, as it can increase photosensitivity.
5. Store the serum in a cool, dark place when not in use.

Variations

- For extra hydration, add a few drops of vitamin E oil to the mixture. Vitamin E is an antioxidant that can help protect the skin from environmental stressors.
- If you have sensitive skin or are concerned about the photosensitizing effects of lemon essential oil, you can substitute it with sweet orange essential oil for a gentler brightening effect.

Storage tips

Keep the serum in a dark, cool place, such as a medicine cabinet or drawer, away from direct sunlight and heat sources to preserve the efficacy of the oils and essential oils.

Tips for allergens

If you are sensitive to any of the essential oils suggested, you can omit them from the recipe. Always perform a patch test on a small area of your skin before using the serum extensively, especially if you have sensitive skin or are prone to allergies.

Castor Oil and Hyaluronic Acid Hydrating Gel

Beneficial effects

The Castor Oil and Hyaluronic Acid Hydrating Gel is designed to provide deep hydration, improve skin elasticity, and reduce the appearance of fine lines and wrinkles. Castor oil, with its rich fatty acid content, nourishes and moisturizes the skin, while hyaluronic acid, known for its ability to hold up to 1000 times its weight in water, plumps and hydrates the skin, resulting in a smoother, more youthful appearance.

Ingredients

- 2 tablespoons of cold-pressed castor oil
- 1 teaspoon of hyaluronic acid powder
- 1/2 cup of distilled water
- 1/4 teaspoon of xanthan gum (as a thickener)
- 5 drops of lavender essential oil (optional for scent and additional skin benefits)

Instructions

1. Begin by dissolving the hyaluronic acid powder in distilled water. Stir well and let it sit for a few hours or until fully hydrated; the mixture will turn into a gel-like consistency.
2. In a separate bowl, mix the xanthan gum with castor oil until the mixture is smooth and uniform.
3. Slowly add the hyaluronic acid gel to the castor oil mixture, stirring continuously to ensure a homogenous blend.
4. If using, add the lavender essential oil to the mixture and stir well.
5. Transfer the hydrating gel into a clean, sterilized jar with a lid.
6. To use, apply a small amount of the gel to your face and neck after cleansing, gently massaging it into the skin in upward motions.

Variations

- For additional anti-aging benefits, mix in a vitamin C serum before applying the gel.
- If you have sensitive skin, omit the lavender essential oil or replace it with chamomile essential oil for its soothing properties.

Storage tips

Store the hydrating gel in a cool, dark place, preferably in the refrigerator, to maintain its freshness and efficacy. Use within 1 month for best results.

Tips for allergens

If you are allergic to lavender or any other essential oils, it's best to omit them from the recipe. Always perform a patch test on a small area of your skin before using the gel extensively to ensure there is no adverse reaction.

Castor Oil and Green Clay Detox Mask

Beneficial effects

The Castor Oil and Green Clay Detox Mask is designed to deeply cleanse and detoxify the skin, drawing out impurities and excess oils that can lead to acne and blemishes. Castor oil, with its antimicrobial and anti-inflammatory properties, soothes the skin and promotes healing, while green clay, rich in minerals, absorbs toxins and tightens pores. This mask leaves the skin refreshed, clear, and with a healthy glow, making it an excellent addition to any skincare routine for those seeking to maintain a radiant and youthful complexion.

Ingredients
-   2 tablespoons of cold-pressed castor oil
-   1 tablespoon of green clay powder
-   3 tablespoons of distilled water (adjust as needed for desired consistency)
-   5 drops of tea tree essential oil (optional for added antimicrobial benefits)

Instructions
1. In a non-metallic bowl, mix the green clay powder with distilled water until a smooth paste is formed.
2. Add the cold-pressed castor oil to the clay mixture and stir until well combined.
3. If using, incorporate the tea tree essential oil into the mixture for its additional antimicrobial and soothing properties.
4. Apply the mask evenly over a clean, dry face, avoiding the eye and mouth areas.
5. Leave the mask on for 10-15 minutes or until it begins to dry but is not completely hardened, as this can draw moisture from the skin.
6. Rinse off the mask with lukewarm water, gently removing all traces of clay and oil.
7. Pat your face dry with a soft towel and follow up with a moisturizer suitable for your skin type.

Variations
-   For dry skin types, add a teaspoon of honey to the mixture for its moisturizing and antibacterial properties.
-   If you have sensitive skin, reduce the amount of tea tree essential oil to 2-3 drops to minimize the risk of irritation.

Storage tips

Prepare this mask fresh each time to ensure the potency and effectiveness of the ingredients. The green clay and castor oil can be stored separately in airtight containers in a cool, dry place for future use.

Tips for allergens

Individuals with sensitivity to tea tree oil can omit it from the recipe or substitute it with lavender essential oil for a gentler alternative that still offers antimicrobial benefits. Always perform a patch test on a small area of your skin before applying the mask extensively, especially if you are incorporating new essential oils into the mix.

Castor Oil and Papaya Enzyme Exfoliating Mask

Beneficial effects

The Castor Oil and Papaya Enzyme Exfoliating Mask combines the deep moisturizing properties of castor oil with the natural exfoliating enzymes found in papaya. This powerful duo works to gently remove dead skin cells, hydrate the skin, and promote a brighter, more even complexion. Papaya enzymes, known as papain, help break down inactive proteins and eliminate skin impurities, while castor oil provides essential fatty acids to nourish and restore the skin's barrier. Suitable for all skin types, this mask can help reduce the appearance of fine lines, dark spots, and provide an overall rejuvenated look.

Ingredients

- 2 tablespoons of cold-pressed castor oil
- 1/2 ripe papaya, mashed
- 1 tablespoon of honey (optional, for additional moisturizing benefits)
- 1 teaspoon of lemon juice (optional, for brightening effects)

Instructions

1. In a clean mixing bowl, combine the mashed papaya and cold-pressed castor oil until you achieve a smooth consistency.
2. If using, stir in the honey for its hydrating properties and lemon juice for its ability to brighten and even out skin tone. Mix well.
3. Apply a generous layer of the mask to clean, dry skin, avoiding the eye area.
4. Leave the mask on for 15-20 minutes, allowing the enzymes and oils to penetrate deeply.
5. Rinse off with lukewarm water, gently patting your skin dry with a soft towel.
6. Follow up with your regular moisturizer to lock in hydration.

Variations

- For sensitive skin, omit the lemon juice as it may cause irritation.
- Add a teaspoon of ground oats to the mixture for a soothing effect and additional gentle exfoliation.

Storage tips

Prepare this mask fresh for each use to ensure the potency of the papaya enzymes and the freshness of the ingredients. It is not recommended to store any leftovers as the natural components quickly lose their effectiveness once mixed.

Tips for allergens

Individuals with latex allergy should be cautious when using papaya, as it contains enzymes similar to those found in latex that can cause reactions. Always perform a patch test on a small area of your arm before applying the mask to your face. If you have a known allergy to honey, you can omit it from the recipe without affecting the mask's exfoliating and moisturizing properties.

Castor Oil and Blueberry Antioxidant Cream

Beneficial effects

The Castor Oil and Blueberry Antioxidant Cream utilizes the hydrating properties of castor oil and the antioxidant benefits of blueberries to create a potent skin-care remedy. This cream is designed to combat oxidative stress and environmental damage to the skin, reducing signs of aging, improving skin texture, and enhancing the skin's natural glow. The ricinoleic acid in castor oil promotes skin health by deeply moisturizing and reducing inflammation, while the antioxidants in blueberries help to repair and protect the skin from damage caused by free radicals.

Ingredients

-   1/4 cup cold-pressed castor oil
-   1/4 cup fresh blueberries
-   1/4 cup shea butter
-   1 tablespoon beeswax
-   1 teaspoon vitamin E oil
-   5 drops lavender essential oil

Instructions

1. In a double boiler, melt the shea butter and beeswax together until fully combined.
2. Puree the blueberries in a blender until smooth. Strain the puree to remove any solid pieces.
3. Once the shea butter and beeswax mixture has melted, remove it from heat and allow it to cool slightly.
4. Stir in the cold-pressed castor oil and blueberry puree into the shea butter and beeswax mixture. Mix thoroughly to ensure all ingredients are well incorporated.
5. Add the vitamin E oil and lavender essential oil to the mixture, stirring well.
6. Pour the cream into a clean jar and allow it to cool and solidify at room temperature.
7. Once solidified, seal the jar. Your antioxidant cream is ready for use.

Variations

-   For added hydration, include a tablespoon of aloe vera gel into the mixture during step 4.
-   If you prefer a vegan option, substitute beeswax with an equal amount of candelilla wax.

Storage tips

Store the cream in a cool, dry place away from direct sunlight. If stored properly, the cream should remain effective for up to 3 months. Ensure the jar is tightly sealed after each use to maintain freshness.

Tips for allergens

If you have sensitive skin or are prone to allergies, perform a patch test on a small area of your skin before applying the cream extensively. Substitute lavender essential oil with chamomile essential oil for a gentler alternative if you're sensitive to lavender.

Castor Oil and Manuka Honey Healing Balm

Beneficial effects

The Castor Oil and Manuka Honey Healing Balm is a powerful combination that leverages the anti-inflammatory and moisturizing properties of castor oil with the antibacterial and healing benefits of Manuka honey. This balm is designed to soothe and heal dry, irritated skin, reduce redness and inflammation, and promote the healing of minor wounds, cuts, and burns. Its natural ingredients make it suitable for sensitive skin, offering a gentle yet effective solution for skin care.

Ingredients

- 1/4 cup cold-pressed castor oil
- 1/4 cup Manuka honey
- 2 tablespoons beeswax pellets
- 1 tablespoon coconut oil
- 5 drops lavender essential oil (optional for additional soothing properties)

Instructions

1. Combine the beeswax pellets and coconut oil in a double boiler over medium heat. Stir continuously until completely melted and combined.
2. Remove from heat and allow to cool slightly before adding the castor oil, blending well.
3. Stir in the Manuka honey until the mixture is uniform.
4. If using, add the lavender essential oil and mix thoroughly.
5. Pour the mixture into a clean, dry container and allow it to cool and solidify.
6. Once cooled, seal the container. Your healing balm is ready for use.

Variations

- For extra skin nourishment, add a teaspoon of vitamin E oil to the mixture.
- To target acne-prone skin, include a few drops of tea tree oil for its antimicrobial properties.

Storage tips

Store the healing balm in a cool, dry place away from direct sunlight. If stored properly, the balm should remain effective and fresh for up to 6 months.

Tips for allergens

If you have a sensitivity or allergy to beeswax, you can substitute it with an equal amount of candelilla wax or soy wax for a vegan-friendly version. Always perform a patch test on a small area of your skin before applying the balm extensively, especially if you have sensitive skin or are prone to allergies.

Castor Oil and Pomegranate Seed Oil Firming Lotion

Beneficial effects

The Castor Oil and Pomegranate Seed Oil Firming Lotion is a luxurious, deeply moisturizing lotion designed to improve skin elasticity and firmness. Castor oil, known for its hydrating and anti-inflammatory properties, works in synergy with pomegranate seed oil, which is rich in antioxidants and punicic acid, to rejuvenate the skin, stimulate collagen production, and protect against signs of aging. This powerful combination helps to smooth fine lines, tighten sagging skin, and provide a youthful glow.

Ingredients

- 1/4 cup cold-pressed castor oil
- 1/4 cup cold-pressed pomegranate seed oil
- 1/4 cup coconut oil
- 1/4 cup shea butter
- 2 tablespoons beeswax
- 10 drops vitamin E oil
- 10 drops lavender essential oil (optional for scent and additional skin benefits)

Instructions

1. Combine coconut oil, shea butter, and beeswax in a double boiler over medium heat. Stir continuously until completely melted and combined.
2. Remove from heat and allow the mixture to cool slightly.
3. Slowly stir in the castor oil and pomegranate seed oil until well blended.
4. Add the vitamin E oil and, if using, the lavender essential oil to the mixture. Stir thoroughly to ensure even distribution.
5. Pour the mixture into a clean, dry container and allow it to cool and solidify at room temperature.
6. Once solidified, seal the container. Your firming lotion is ready to use.

Variations

- For additional anti-aging benefits, include a few drops of rosehip seed oil in the mixture.
- If you prefer a vegan option, use candelilla wax in place of beeswax.

Storage tips

Store your firming lotion in a cool, dry place away from direct sunlight. If stored properly, the lotion should remain effective and fresh for up to 6 months. Ensure the container is tightly sealed to maintain the lotion's potency.

Tips for allergens

If you have sensitivities to coconut oil or shea butter, you can substitute them with mango butter or jojoba oil, which are gentle on the skin and provide similar moisturizing benefits. Always perform a patch test on a small area of your skin before applying the lotion extensively, especially if you have sensitive skin or are prone to allergies.

Castor Oil and Cucumber Hydrating Mist

Beneficial effects

The Castor Oil and Cucumber Hydrating Mist offers a refreshing and hydrating experience for the skin, combining the moisturizing benefits of castor oil with the soothing and cooling properties of cucumber. This mist is ideal for calming irritated or sun-exposed skin, providing a quick moisture boost throughout the day, and helping to maintain a balanced and radiant complexion.

Ingredients

- 1/4 cup distilled water
- 2 tablespoons cold-pressed castor oil
- 1/2 cucumber, blended and strained to extract juice
- 10 drops of lavender essential oil (optional for additional soothing effects)
- Small spray bottle

Instructions

1. In a blender, puree the cucumber until smooth.
2. Using a fine mesh strainer or cheesecloth, strain the cucumber to obtain the juice. You should have approximately 1/4 cup of cucumber juice.
3. In a small bowl, combine the cucumber juice, distilled water, and castor oil. Stir well to mix.
4. If using, add the lavender essential oil to the mixture and stir again to ensure it's evenly distributed.
5. Carefully pour the mixture into a clean, small spray bottle using a funnel if necessary.
6. To use, shake the bottle well before each application to ensure the oil is mixed. Close your eyes and mist your face lightly, holding the bottle about 6 inches away. Allow it to air dry or gently pat the skin with a clean cloth.
7. Apply as needed throughout the day for a refreshing and hydrating boost.

Variations

- For extra cooling effects, store the mist in the refrigerator before use.
- Substitute lavender essential oil with rose or chamomile essential oil for different therapeutic benefits and fragrances.

Storage tips

Store your hydrating mist in the refrigerator to maintain freshness and enhance the cooling effect upon application. Use within 1 week for best quality.

Tips for allergens

If you have sensitive skin or are allergic to any of the essential oils, you can omit them from the recipe. Always perform a patch test on a small area of your skin before using the mist extensively.

Castor Oil and Licorice Root Brightening Cream

Beneficial effects

The Castor Oil and Licorice Root Brightening Cream is crafted to lighten dark spots and even out skin tone, leveraging the natural properties of licorice root, known for its ability to inhibit the enzyme responsible for melanin production. Combined with the hydrating and anti-inflammatory benefits of castor oil, this cream promotes a brighter, more radiant complexion while soothing and moisturizing the skin.

Ingredients

- 2 tablespoons cold-pressed castor oil
- 1 tablespoon licorice root extract
- 1/4 cup shea butter
- 1/4 cup aloe vera gel
- 10 drops of vitamin E oil
- 5 drops of lemon essential oil (optional for added brightening effects)

Instructions

1. In a double boiler, gently melt the shea butter until it's completely liquid.
2. Remove from heat and let it cool for a few minutes.
3. Stir in the cold-pressed castor oil and licorice root extract until well combined.
4. Add the aloe vera gel to the mixture, stirring continuously to ensure a smooth consistency.
5. Mix in the vitamin E oil, and if using, add the lemon essential oil for enhanced skin brightening benefits.
6. Pour the mixture into a clean, dry container and allow it to cool and solidify.
7. Once solidified, seal the container. Your brightening cream is ready for use.

Variations

- For sensitive skin, omit the lemon essential oil as it can be irritating to some skin types.
- If you prefer a vegan option, ensure that the vitamin E oil is sourced from plant-based ingredients.

Storage tips

Store your brightening cream in a cool, dark place to preserve its potency. If stored properly, the cream should remain effective for up to 3 months.

Tips for allergens

If you have a sensitivity to lemon or any citrus-based essential oils, it's best to omit them from the recipe. Always perform a patch test on a small area of your skin before applying the cream extensively, especially if you have sensitive skin or are prone to allergies.

Castor Oil and Oatmeal Soothing Mask

Beneficial effects

The Castor Oil and Oatmeal Soothing Mask combines the deeply hydrating and anti-inflammatory properties of castor oil with the soothing, exfoliating benefits of oatmeal. This natural remedy is designed to moisturize dry, irritated skin, reduce redness, and gently remove dead skin cells, leaving the skin feeling soft, refreshed, and rejuvenated. It's particularly beneficial for those with sensitive or acne-prone skin, as both ingredients are gentle and known for their healing properties.

Ingredients

- 2 tablespoons of cold-pressed castor oil
- 1/3 cup of finely ground oatmeal
- 1/4 cup of warm water
- 1 tablespoon of honey (optional for added moisture and antibacterial properties)

Instructions

1. In a small bowl, mix the finely ground oatmeal with warm water to form a paste.
2. Add the cold-pressed castor oil to the oatmeal paste and stir until well combined.
3. If using, incorporate the honey into the mixture for additional hydration and its antibacterial benefits.
4. Apply the mask evenly over a clean, damp face, avoiding the eye area.
5. Leave the mask on for about 15-20 minutes, allowing the ingredients to nourish and soothe the skin.
6. Rinse off the mask with lukewarm water, gently massaging in a circular motion to exfoliate as you wash it away.
7. Pat your face dry with a soft towel and follow up with your regular moisturizer.

Variations

- For extra calming effects, add a few drops of lavender essential oil to the mixture. Lavender will enhance the soothing properties and add a relaxing scent.
- If you have oily skin, substitute water with green tea to add antioxidant benefits and help balance oil production.

Storage tips

This mask is best used fresh due to the natural ingredients. However, if you have leftover mixture, you can store it in an airtight container in the refrigerator for up to 2 days. Ensure to stir the mixture well before reapplying.

Tips for allergens

If you're sensitive to gluten, ensure to use gluten-free oatmeal to prevent any allergic reactions. For those allergic to honey, you can omit this ingredient or substitute it with aloe vera gel for a similar moisturizing effect without the allergens.

Hair Care Recipes

Castor Oil and Aloe Vera Hair Mask

Beneficial effects
The Castor Oil and Aloe Vera Hair Mask is formulated to deeply nourish and hydrate the scalp and hair, promoting hair growth and reducing dandruff. Castor oil, rich in omega-6 fatty acids, penetrates the hair follicles to stimulate growth and enhance hair health. Aloe Vera, known for its soothing and moisturizing properties, helps to condition the hair, reduce scalp irritation, and provide a natural shine. Together, these ingredients create a powerful hair mask that strengthens and revitalizes the hair from root to tip.

Ingredients
- 3 tablespoons of cold-pressed castor oil
- 2 tablespoons of pure aloe vera gel
- 1 teaspoon of honey (optional for extra hydration)
- 2 drops of rosemary essential oil (optional for stimulating hair growth)

Instructions
1. In a clean bowl, mix the castor oil and aloe vera gel until you achieve a smooth consistency.
2. If using, add the honey to the mixture for additional moisture and the rosemary essential oil to stimulate hair growth. Stir well to combine all the ingredients.
3. Apply the mask evenly to your scalp and hair, working it through from roots to ends.
4. Cover your hair with a shower cap and leave the mask on for at least 30 minutes, or for optimal results, leave it overnight.
5. Rinse the mask out with lukewarm water and shampoo as usual.
6. Repeat this treatment once a week for best results.

Variations
- For dry hair, add an extra tablespoon of honey to the mixture to enhance moisture.
- If you have oily hair, reduce the amount of castor oil to 2 tablespoons and add a tablespoon of lemon juice to balance the scalp's oil production.

Storage tips
Prepare this hair mask fresh each time to ensure the potency of the ingredients. The individual components, castor oil and aloe vera gel, should be stored in cool, dry places. Castor oil can be kept in a cupboard away from direct sunlight, while aloe vera gel, especially if natural, should be refrigerated.

Tips for allergens
If you're sensitive to honey or essential oils, you can omit these ingredients from the recipe. Always perform a patch test on a small section of your scalp before applying the mask entirely, especially if you're incorporating new ingredients into your hair care routine.

Castor Oil and Argan Oil Shine Serum

Beneficial effects

The Castor Oil and Argan Oil Shine Serum is a luxurious blend designed to nourish and add a luminous shine to your hair. Castor oil, renowned for its ability to promote hair growth and scalp health, works in harmony with argan oil, known as 'liquid gold' for its high content of antioxidants, essential fatty acids, and vitamin E. Together, they create a powerful serum that not only strengthens and protects your hair from environmental damage but also leaves it silky, shiny, and smooth.

Ingredients

- 2 tablespoons of cold-pressed castor oil
- 2 tablespoons of cold-pressed argan oil
- 5 drops of rosemary essential oil (optional for stimulating hair growth and adding a refreshing scent)
- Small glass bottle with dropper

Instructions

1. In a small bowl, mix together the castor oil and argan oil until well combined.
2. If using, add the rosemary essential oil to the oil blend and stir thoroughly. The rosemary essential oil is optional but recommended for its ability to stimulate hair growth and its refreshing scent.
3. Carefully pour the mixture into the glass dropper bottle.
4. To use, apply a few drops of the serum to the palm of your hand, rub your hands together to warm the oil, and then gently work it through the ends of your damp or dry hair. Avoid applying too much product near the roots to prevent greasiness.
5. Style your hair as usual. The serum can be used daily or as needed to add shine and moisture to your hair.

Variations

- For added moisture, include a few drops of vitamin E oil to the mixture. Vitamin E oil can help repair damaged hair follicles and encourage healthy hair growth.
- If you have fine hair, reduce the amount of castor oil to 1 tablespoon and increase the argan oil to 3 tablespoons for a lighter serum that won't weigh your hair down.

Storage tips

Store your shine serum in a cool, dark place to preserve the potency of the oils. The dark glass dropper bottle helps protect the oils from light, extending their shelf life. If stored properly, the serum should remain effective for up to 6 months.

Tips for allergens

If you are sensitive to rosemary or any other essential oils, you can omit them from the recipe. Always perform a patch test on a small area of your skin or scalp before using the serum extensively, especially if you have sensitive skin or are prone to allergies.

Castor Oil and Biotin Hair Strengthener

Beneficial effects

The Castor Oil and Biotin Hair Strengthener is a potent formulation designed to nourish the scalp, strengthen hair follicles, and promote healthy hair growth. Castor oil, rich in omega-6 fatty acids, penetrates deep into the hair follicles, providing moisture and encouraging thicker hair growth. Biotin, a B-vitamin, plays a crucial role in the health of the hair, skin, and nails, supporting hair growth and reducing hair loss. Together, this combination helps to fortify the hair from the roots, making it less prone to breakage and giving it a fuller, healthier appearance.

Ingredients

- 3 tablespoons of cold-pressed castor oil
- 2 capsules of biotin (powder form)
- 1 tablespoon of coconut oil
- 5 drops of rosemary essential oil

Instructions

1. In a small bowl, mix the cold-pressed castor oil and coconut oil.
2. Carefully open the biotin capsules and add the powder to the oil mixture.
3. Add the rosemary essential oil to the bowl and stir all the ingredients until well combined.
4. Apply the mixture directly to the scalp and through the length of your hair, focusing on areas that are thinning or prone to breakage.
5. Massage the scalp gently for a few minutes to improve circulation and ensure the mixture is evenly distributed.
6. Leave the treatment in your hair for at least an hour or, for best results, overnight.
7. Wash your hair with a gentle shampoo and condition as usual.

Variations

- For dry hair, add a teaspoon of honey to the mixture for additional moisture.
- If you have oily hair, reduce the amount of coconut oil to avoid making your hair greasy.

Storage tips

Prepare this mixture fresh each time to ensure the potency of the biotin and the essential oils. It's best not to store any leftovers as the biotin may lose its effectiveness when exposed to air for extended periods.

Tips for allergens

If you're allergic to coconut oil, you can substitute it with jojoba oil, which is hypoallergenic and also beneficial for hair strength and growth. Always conduct a patch test on your skin before applying the mixture to your scalp, especially if you're using rosemary essential oil for the first time, to ensure there's no allergic reaction.

Castor Oil and Hibiscus Hair Rinse

Beneficial effects

The Castor Oil and Hibiscus Hair Rinse leverages the potent moisturizing properties of castor oil and the natural benefits of hibiscus to create a hair care solution that promotes a healthy scalp and vibrant, lustrous hair. This rinse aids in restoring the scalp's natural oil balance, encouraging hair growth, and providing antioxidants that protect hair from damage. Hibiscus is known for its ability to enhance hair color and shine, while castor oil strengthens and conditions the hair, reducing breakage and promoting hair thickness.

Ingredients

- 1/4 cup of cold-pressed castor oil
- 1 cup of water
- 1/2 cup of fresh hibiscus petals or 2 tablespoons of dried hibiscus petals
- 1 tablespoon of apple cider vinegar (optional for added shine and pH balance)

Instructions

1. Boil the water in a small pot and add the hibiscus petals. Reduce the heat and simmer for 15-20 minutes to allow the petals to infuse the water.
2. Strain the hibiscus water into a bowl, removing the petals. Let the water cool to room temperature.
3. Once cooled, add the cold-pressed castor oil to the hibiscus water. If using, incorporate the apple cider vinegar into the mixture.
4. Transfer the hair rinse to a clean bottle for easy application.
5. After shampooing and conditioning your hair as usual, slowly pour the Castor Oil and Hibiscus Hair Rinse over your scalp and hair as a final rinse. Do not rinse out.
6. Gently massage the scalp for a few minutes to ensure the mixture is evenly distributed throughout your hair.
7. Style your hair as usual.

Variations

- For an extra moisturizing boost, add a teaspoon of honey to the mixture. Honey is a natural humectant that helps retain moisture in the hair.
- To address scalp issues such as itchiness or dandruff, include a few drops of tea tree essential oil for its antifungal and antibacterial properties.

Storage tips

Prepare this rinse fresh for each use to ensure the potency of the nutrients. If you have leftover hibiscus water, it can be stored in the refrigerator for up to a week. Ensure any containers used for storage are clean and airtight.

Tips for allergens

If you have sensitivity to hibiscus, perform a patch test on your skin before applying the rinse to your scalp and hair. For those allergic to apple cider vinegar, it can be omitted from the recipe without compromising the rinse's benefits.

Castor Oil and Lavender Hair Serum

Beneficial effects

The Castor Oil and Lavender Hair Serum is designed to nourish and strengthen hair, promote hair growth, and improve scalp health. Castor oil is renowned for its ability to enhance hair thickness and growth due to its high content of ricinoleic acid, while lavender oil is celebrated for its soothing properties and ability to reduce scalp inflammation, dandruff, and balance sebum production. Together, they create a potent serum that not only fosters a healthy scalp environment conducive to hair growth but also leaves hair looking shiny, feeling soft, and smelling delightful.

Ingredients

- 3 tablespoons of cold-pressed castor oil
- 5 drops of lavender essential oil
- 2 tablespoons of jojoba oil (as a carrier oil to dilute the mixture and enhance application)
- Small glass bottle with dropper

Instructions

1. In a clean bowl, combine the castor oil and jojoba oil. These oils serve as the base of your serum, providing deep moisturization and facilitating easier application.
2. Add the lavender essential oil to the oil mixture. Lavender oil not only adds a calming scent but also brings its scalp health benefits to the serum.
3. Stir the oils together until they are well blended.
4. Using a funnel, carefully pour the serum into the glass bottle. The dropper will help in applying the serum directly to the scalp and hair.
5. To apply, use the dropper to distribute the serum evenly across the scalp and through the hair, focusing on areas of concern such as thinning edges or dry ends.
6. Massage the serum into the scalp for a few minutes to stimulate blood circulation and ensure the oils are absorbed.
7. Leave the serum in your hair for at least 30 minutes or overnight for deep conditioning. Wash hair as usual afterward.

Variations

- For an extra boost of growth and scalp health, add 2 drops of rosemary essential oil to the mixture. Rosemary is known to stimulate hair growth and improve hair thickness.
- If you have dry hair, consider adding a tablespoon of sweet almond oil to the serum for additional hydration.

Storage tips

Store the serum in a cool, dark place to preserve the integrity of the essential oils. The dark glass bottle helps protect the oils from light, which can degrade their quality over time. When stored properly, the serum should remain effective for up to 6 months.

Tips for allergens

If you are sensitive to lavender or any other essential oils, you can omit them from the recipe. Always perform a patch test on a small area of your skin before applying the serum extensively, especially if you have sensitive skin or are prone to allergies.

Castor Oil and Peppermint Scalp Treatment

Beneficial effects

The Castor Oil and Peppermint Scalp Treatment is designed to stimulate hair growth, soothe scalp irritation, and provide a refreshing, cooling sensation. Castor oil, rich in ricinoleic acid, enhances blood circulation to the scalp, promoting healthier hair growth, while peppermint oil's menthol content offers a cooling effect that soothes itchiness and dandruff, making this treatment ideal for those looking to improve scalp health and encourage hair growth.

Ingredients

- 3 tablespoons of cold-pressed castor oil
- 5 drops of peppermint essential oil
- 2 tablespoons of coconut oil (as a carrier oil to dilute the mixture)

Instructions

1. In a small bowl, mix the cold-pressed castor oil with coconut oil thoroughly. Coconut oil is used to dilute the potent castor oil and peppermint oil, making the mixture gentler on the scalp.
2. Add the peppermint essential oil to the castor and coconut oil mixture, and stir well to ensure the oils are evenly blended.
3. Apply the oil mixture directly to the scalp with your fingertips, massaging gently in circular motions. Focus on areas that are particularly dry or where hair thinning is noticeable.
4. Leave the treatment on for at least 30 minutes, or for enhanced benefits, cover your hair with a shower cap and leave it on overnight.
5. Wash your hair thoroughly with a gentle shampoo to remove the oil. It may require two washes to completely remove the oil residue.
6. For best results, use this treatment once or twice a week.

Variations

- For an extra moisturizing effect, add 1 tablespoon of honey to the mixture. Honey is a natural humectant that can help to lock in moisture.
- If you have sensitive skin, reduce the amount of peppermint essential oil to 2-3 drops to minimize the risk of irritation.

Storage tips

Prepare the mixture fresh each time before use to ensure the potency of the essential oils. If you must prepare in advance, store the oil blend in an airtight container in a cool, dark place for up to one week.

Tips for allergens

If you're sensitive to peppermint oil, you can substitute it with rosemary essential oil, which also promotes scalp circulation and hair growth, without the intense cooling effect. Always perform a patch test on a small area of your skin before applying the treatment to your scalp, especially if you're using new essential oils for the first time.

Castor Oil and Rice Water Hair Rinse

Beneficial effects

The Castor Oil and Rice Water Hair Rinse leverages the nourishing and fortifying properties of castor oil along with the strengthening and smoothing benefits of rice water. This combination promotes hair growth, improves hair elasticity, and adds a natural sheen, making it an excellent treatment for those seeking to revitalize their hair and scalp health.

Ingredients

- 1/4 cup cold-pressed castor oil
- 1 cup rice water (fermented for added benefits)
- 5 drops of lavender essential oil (optional for scent and scalp health)

Instructions

1. Prepare rice water by rinsing 1/2 cup of uncooked rice to remove any impurities. Soak the rice in 2 cups of water for 24 hours at room temperature to ferment and release its nutrients. Strain the rice water into a bowl and set aside.
2. In a mixing bowl, combine the castor oil with 1 cup of the prepared rice water. Stir well to ensure the mixture is well blended.
3. If using, add the lavender essential oil to the mixture for its calming properties and pleasant scent. Mix thoroughly.
4. After shampooing your hair, slowly pour the castor oil and rice water rinse over your scalp and hair, ensuring even coverage.
5. Massage the mixture into your scalp for a few minutes to stimulate blood circulation and ensure the nutrients are absorbed.
6. Leave the rinse on your hair for 5-10 minutes to allow the beneficial properties to penetrate deeply.
7. Rinse your hair thoroughly with cool water. For best results, use this treatment once a week to enhance hair growth and texture.

Variations

- For dry or damaged hair, add a tablespoon of honey to the mixture for its moisturizing properties.
- If dealing with scalp issues like dandruff, include a few drops of tea tree essential oil for its antifungal and antibacterial benefits.

Storage tips

The rice water should be used immediately after preparation for the best results. Any leftover rice water can be stored in the refrigerator for up to a week. Ensure the castor oil is kept in a cool, dark place to maintain its potency.

Tips for allergens

If you're sensitive to essential oils, you can omit them from the recipe. Always perform a patch test on your skin before applying the rinse extensively, especially if you're incorporating new ingredients into your hair care routine.

Castor Oil and Shea Butter Deep Conditioner

Beneficial effects

The Castor Oil and Shea Butter Deep Conditioner is a luxurious, deeply nourishing treatment designed to restore moisture, enhance hair elasticity, and reduce frizz. By combining the hydrating properties of castor oil with the rich, emollient benefits of shea butter, this conditioner penetrates deeply into the hair shaft, replenishing lost oils and locking in moisture. It's particularly beneficial for those with dry, brittle, or damaged hair, promoting a healthier, smoother, and more manageable mane.

Ingredients

- 3 tablespoons cold-pressed castor oil
- 2 tablespoons shea butter
- 1 tablespoon coconut oil
- 1 teaspoon honey (optional for additional moisture and shine)
- 5 drops of lavender essential oil (optional for scent and scalp health)

Instructions

1. Start by melting the shea butter and coconut oil together in a double boiler over low heat until completely liquid.
2. Remove from heat and allow the mixture to cool slightly before stirring in the cold-pressed castor oil. Mix thoroughly to ensure the oils are well blended.
3. If using, add the honey and lavender essential oil to the oil mixture and stir until evenly distributed.
4. Apply the deep conditioner to clean, damp hair, focusing on the ends and working your way up to the scalp. Ensure that every strand is coated.
5. Cover your hair with a shower cap and let the conditioner sit for at least 30 minutes. For deeper conditioning, leave it on for up to an hour.
6. Rinse the conditioner out thoroughly with warm water, then shampoo and condition as usual.

Variations

- For an extra protein boost, add 1 tablespoon of Greek yogurt to the mixture. Protein helps to strengthen hair strands and prevent breakage.
- If you have very fine hair, you can reduce the amount of shea butter to 1 tablespoon to prevent weighing down your hair.

Storage tips

Prepare this deep conditioner fresh for each use to ensure the maximum benefit from the natural ingredients. It's not recommended to store any leftovers due to the inclusion of fresh components like honey, which may not preserve well.

Tips for allergens

If you're allergic to coconut oil, you can substitute it with jojoba oil or almond oil, both of which are also excellent for hair health and hydration. Always perform a patch test on a small section of your scalp before applying the mixture entirely, especially if you decide to add essential oils, to ensure there is no adverse reaction.

Castor Oil and Tea Tree Oil Scalp Soother

Beneficial effects

The Castor Oil and Tea Tree Oil Scalp Soother is a natural remedy designed to alleviate scalp irritation, dandruff, and promote a healthy hair growth environment. Castor oil, with its antibacterial and moisturizing properties, helps to soothe the scalp and lock in moisture, while tea tree oil's antifungal capabilities target dandruff and dryness. This combination not only helps to relieve discomfort but also fosters a healthy scalp, leading to stronger and healthier hair growth.

Ingredients

- 3 tablespoons of cold-pressed castor oil
- 10 drops of tea tree essential oil
- 2 tablespoons of coconut oil (as a carrier and for additional hydration)

Instructions

1. Begin by warming the coconut oil in a small bowl until it becomes liquid. Ensure it's warm, not hot, to maintain the integrity of the oils.
2. Add the cold-pressed castor oil to the warmed coconut oil, mixing thoroughly to combine.
3. Incorporate the tea tree essential oil into the oil blend, stirring well to ensure an even distribution.
4. Apply the mixture directly to the scalp, using your fingertips to massage it in gently. Focus on areas that are particularly dry or irritated.
5. Allow the treatment to sit on the scalp for at least 30 minutes, though leaving it on overnight under a shower cap can provide enhanced benefits.
6. Wash the treatment out with a gentle shampoo, ensuring all oil is removed from the scalp and hair.
7. Repeat this treatment once or twice a week for best results.

Variations

- For an extra soothing effect, add 5 drops of lavender essential oil to the mixture. Lavender will not only enhance the scent but also add calming properties to soothe the scalp further.
- If your scalp is extremely sensitive, reduce the amount of tea tree oil to 5 drops to minimize the risk of irritation.

Storage tips
Prepare this mixture fresh each time to ensure the potency of the essential oils. If you must prepare in advance, store the blend in a dark glass bottle in a cool, dark place for up to one month.

Tips for allergens
If you have a known allergy to coconut oil, you can substitute it with jojoba oil, which is hypoallergenic and also beneficial for scalp health. Always perform a patch test on a small area of your skin before applying the treatment extensively, especially if you are incorporating new essential oils into your routine.

Castor Oil and Vitamin E Hair Repair Serum

Beneficial effects
The Castor Oil and Vitamin E Hair Repair Serum is specifically formulated to restore vitality and shine to damaged, dry, and brittle hair. Castor oil, rich in omega-9 fatty acids, penetrates the hair shaft, promoting growth and repairing split ends, while Vitamin E provides antioxidant protection against environmental stressors, preventing further damage. This serum revitalizes the scalp, encourages healthy hair growth, and leaves hair soft, glossy, and smooth.

Ingredients
- 3 tablespoons of cold-pressed castor oil
- 1 tablespoon of Vitamin E oil
- 5 drops of rosemary essential oil (optional for stimulating hair growth)
- Small glass bottle with dropper

Instructions
1. In a small bowl, mix the castor oil and Vitamin E oil until well combined.
2. If using, add the rosemary essential oil to the mixture for its hair growth-stimulating properties. Stir thoroughly.
3. Carefully pour the oil blend into the glass bottle using a small funnel.
4. To apply, use the dropper to dispense a few drops of the serum directly onto your scalp and hair ends.
5. Massage gently into the scalp with your fingertips in circular motions for a few minutes to enhance absorption and stimulate blood flow.
6. Leave the serum in your hair for at least 30 minutes or overnight for deep conditioning.
7. Wash your hair with a gentle shampoo and condition as usual.

Variations
- For added moisture, include a few drops of argan oil in the mixture.
- If you have fine or oily hair, reduce the amount of castor oil to 2 tablespoons to prevent weighing down your hair.

Storage tips

Store the serum in a cool, dark place to maintain the potency of the oils. The dark glass bottle will help protect the oils from light degradation. Ensure the bottle is tightly sealed to prevent oxidation. The serum should remain fresh and effective for up to 6 months.

Tips for allergens

If you're sensitive to rosemary or any essential oils, you can omit them from the recipe. Always perform a patch test on a small area of your scalp or skin before using the serum extensively, especially if you have sensitive skin or are prone to allergies.

Body Care Recipes

Castor Oil and Cocoa Butter Body Lotion

Beneficial effects
The Castor Oil and Cocoa Butter Body Lotion is a deeply hydrating and nourishing formula designed to moisturize dry skin, improve skin elasticity, and reduce the appearance of scars and stretch marks. Castor oil, rich in ricinoleic acid, has anti-inflammatory properties that soothe irritated skin, while cocoa butter, packed with fatty acids, provides a barrier that locks in moisture and improves skin health. This combination results in a luxurious lotion that leaves skin feeling soft, supple, and rejuvenated.

Ingredients
- 1/4 cup cold-pressed castor oil
- 1/4 cup cocoa butter
- 1/4 cup coconut oil
- 2 tablespoons beeswax
- 10 drops of lavender essential oil (optional for scent and additional skin benefits)

Instructions
1. Combine cocoa butter, coconut oil, and beeswax in a double boiler over medium heat. Stir continuously until completely melted and combined.
2. Remove from heat and let the mixture cool slightly.
3. Stir in the cold-pressed castor oil until well blended.
4. If using, add the lavender essential oil to the mixture and stir thoroughly.
5. Pour the mixture into a clean, dry container and allow it to cool and solidify at room temperature.
6. Once solidified, seal the container. Your body lotion is ready to use.

Variations
- For extra hydration, add a tablespoon of almond oil to the mixture.
- If you prefer a vegan option, substitute beeswax with an equal amount of candelilla wax or soy wax.

Storage tips
Store your body lotion in a cool, dry place away from direct sunlight. If stored properly, the lotion should remain effective and fresh for up to 6 months. Ensure the container is tightly sealed to maintain the lotion's potency.

Tips for allergens
If you are sensitive to coconut oil, you can substitute it with jojoba oil, which is also nourishing and less likely to cause irritation. Always perform a patch test on a small area of your skin before applying the lotion extensively, especially if you have sensitive skin or are prone to allergies.

Castor Oil and Epsom Salt Bath Soak

Beneficial effects

The Castor Oil and Epsom Salt Bath Soak is a therapeutic remedy designed to soothe sore muscles, hydrate the skin, and promote relaxation. The combination of castor oil and Epsom salt works synergistically to reduce inflammation, relieve pain, and detoxify the body. Castor oil's ricinoleic acid has anti-inflammatory properties that, when absorbed through the skin, can help alleviate muscle tension and discomfort. Epsom salt, rich in magnesium, aids in relaxing muscle cramps and improving circulation. This bath soak is perfect for unwinding after a long day and is especially beneficial for those seeking a natural way to address body aches and skin dryness.

Ingredients

- 1/4 cup cold-pressed castor oil
- 2 cups Epsom salt
- 10 drops lavender essential oil (optional for a calming scent)
- Warm bath water

Instructions

1. Fill your bathtub with warm water, ensuring it's at a comfortable temperature for soaking.
2. While the tub is filling, in a small bowl, mix the cold-pressed castor oil with the Epsom salt. Stir well to ensure the oil is evenly distributed throughout the salt.
3. If using, add the lavender essential oil to the Epsom salt and castor oil mixture. Mix thoroughly to combine.
4. Once the bathtub is filled, pour the mixture into the water and use your hand to swirl the water, helping the salt dissolve and the oil disperse evenly.
5. Step into the bath and soak for at least 20 minutes, allowing your body to absorb the minerals and the oil.
6. After soaking, gently pat your skin dry with a towel to avoid removing the moisturizing layer of castor oil on your skin.

Variations

- For additional detoxification benefits, add 1/2 cup of baking soda to the mixture. Baking soda helps in drawing out toxins and leaving the skin feeling soft.
- If you prefer a more invigorating scent, substitute lavender essential oil with peppermint or eucalyptus essential oil, which can also help in relieving nasal congestion and promoting clear breathing.

Storage tips

Prepare the soak mixture fresh for each bath to ensure the best results. Store any unused castor oil and Epsom salt in a cool, dry place for future use. Essential oils should be kept in dark, airtight containers to preserve their potency.

Tips for allergens

If you are sensitive to lavender or any other essential oils, you can omit them from the recipe. Always conduct a patch test on your forearm with the diluted essential oil before adding it to your bath, especially if you have sensitive skin or are prone to allergies.

Castor Oil and Shea Butter Body Butter

Beneficial effects

The Castor Oil and Shea Butter Body Butter is a deeply moisturizing and healing treatment designed to soothe dry, irritated skin, and restore elasticity. This rich body butter combines the anti-inflammatory properties of castor oil with the intense moisturizing capabilities of shea butter, making it an ideal remedy for those seeking to nourish and rejuvenate their skin. It's particularly effective for areas prone to dryness like elbows, knees, and heels, as well as for conditions such as eczema and psoriasis.

Ingredients

- 1/2 cup cold-pressed castor oil
- 1/2 cup raw shea butter
- 1/4 cup coconut oil
- 1/4 cup almond oil
- 10 drops of lavender essential oil (optional for scent and additional skin-soothing benefits)

Instructions

1. In a double boiler, gently melt the shea butter and coconut oil together until fully liquid.
2. Remove from heat and let the mixture cool slightly before adding the castor oil and almond oil. Stir well to combine.
3. Once the mixture has cooled to room temperature but before it solidifies, add the lavender essential oil if using, and mix thoroughly.
4. Pour the mixture into a clean, dry container and allow it to cool and solidify completely. You can place it in the refrigerator to speed up this process.
5. Once solidified, use a hand mixer to whip the body butter until it reaches a light and fluffy consistency.
6. Transfer the whipped body butter into airtight jars for storage.

Variations

- For extra dry skin, add a tablespoon of vitamin E oil to the mixture for its healing properties.
- Customize the scent by using different essential oils such as rose, geranium, or ylang-ylang, which also offer various skin benefits.

Storage tips

Store the body butter in a cool, dry place away from direct sunlight. If stored properly in an airtight container, it can last for up to 6 months. During warmer months, you may want to keep it in the refrigerator to maintain its firmness.

Tips for allergens

For those with nut allergies, you can substitute almond oil with jojoba oil or olive oil. Always perform a patch test on a small area of your skin before applying the body butter extensively, especially if you have sensitive skin or are prone to allergies.

Castor Oil and Lavender Body Scrub

Beneficial effects

The Castor Oil and Lavender Body Scrub combines the powerful moisturizing properties of castor oil with the soothing and aromatic benefits of lavender. This scrub is designed to gently exfoliate the skin, removing dead skin cells and promoting the regeneration of new cells. The castor oil deeply hydrates, leaving the skin feeling soft and smooth, while the lavender provides a calming effect, reducing stress and promoting relaxation. This scrub is perfect for rejuvenating the skin, making it an ideal addition to any self-care routine.

Ingredients

- 1/2 cup cold-pressed castor oil
- 1 cup granulated sugar
- 1/4 cup almond oil
- 10-15 drops lavender essential oil
- 2 tablespoons dried lavender buds

Instructions

1. In a medium-sized mixing bowl, combine the granulated sugar with the cold-pressed castor oil and almond oil. Stir until the oils are well incorporated into the sugar, creating a uniform mixture.
2. Add the lavender essential oil to the mixture, adjusting the amount based on your scent preference. Mix thoroughly to ensure the essential oil is evenly distributed throughout the scrub.
3. Gently fold in the dried lavender buds, adding a natural, exfoliating texture and enhancing the scrub's aromatic properties.
4. Transfer the scrub into a clean, dry jar with a secure lid.
5. To use, apply a generous amount of the body scrub to damp skin in the shower or bath. Gently massage in circular motions, focusing on rough areas such as elbows, knees, and heels. Rinse off with warm water.

Variations

- For a sugar-free version, substitute the granulated sugar with fine sea salt, which offers a different texture and mineral benefits for the skin.
- If you have sensitive skin, replace almond oil with jojoba oil, which is lighter and less likely to cause irritation.

Storage tips
Store the body scrub in an airtight container at room temperature, away from direct sunlight. The scrub should remain fresh and effective for up to 3 months. Ensure the lid is tightly closed after each use to prevent moisture from entering the jar.

Tips for allergens
If you're allergic to almond oil, substituting it with coconut oil or olive oil can provide similar moisturizing benefits without the risk of an allergic reaction. Always perform a patch test on a small area of your skin before using the scrub extensively, especially if you're incorporating new ingredients into your skincare routine.

Castor Oil and Aloe Vera Body Gel

Beneficial effects
The Castor Oil and Aloe Vera Body Gel is a soothing, hydrating treatment designed to moisturize and heal dry, irritated skin. Castor oil's anti-inflammatory properties work to soothe skin irritations and promote healing, while aloe vera's natural enzymes and vitamins nourish and hydrate the skin, improving its overall texture and elasticity. This gel is perfect for after-sun care, reducing redness and discomfort from sunburn, or as a daily moisturizer for a soft, smooth complexion.

Ingredients
- 1/4 cup cold-pressed castor oil
- 3/4 cup pure aloe vera gel
- 10 drops of lavender essential oil (optional for calming scent and additional skin benefits)
- Small glass jar or bottle for storage

Instructions
1. In a clean bowl, mix the cold-pressed castor oil with the aloe vera gel until you achieve a smooth, consistent texture.
2. If using, add the lavender essential oil to the mixture and stir well to ensure it's evenly distributed.
3. Carefully pour the body gel into a clean, dry glass jar or bottle.
4. To apply, gently massage a small amount of the gel onto the skin until fully absorbed. Focus on areas that are particularly dry or irritated.
5. Use daily after showering or as needed throughout the day for a refreshing moisture boost.

Variations
- For extra cooling effects, store the gel in the refrigerator before use. The chilled gel will provide a soothing sensation, especially beneficial for sunburned or inflamed skin.
- To address specific skin concerns, such as acne or signs of aging, substitute lavender essential oil with tea tree oil for its antimicrobial properties or rosehip oil for its anti-aging benefits.

Storage tips

Store the Castor Oil and Aloe Vera Body Gel in a cool, dark place to maintain its freshness and efficacy. If refrigerated, the gel can last for up to one month. Ensure the container is tightly sealed to prevent contamination.

Tips for allergens

If you have sensitive skin or are allergic to lavender, you can omit the essential oil or substitute it with another skin-friendly essential oil like chamomile or frankincense. Always perform a patch test on a small area of your skin before applying the gel extensively.

Castor Oil and Chamomile Body Wash

Beneficial effects

The Castor Oil and Chamomile Body Wash is a gentle, soothing formula designed to cleanse the skin while providing deep hydration and reducing inflammation. Ideal for sensitive or dry skin, this body wash combines the moisturizing properties of castor oil with the calming effects of chamomile, resulting in a soft, nourished complexion. Regular use can help soothe skin irritations, reduce redness, and promote a more even skin tone.

Ingredients

- 1/4 cup cold-pressed castor oil
- 1/4 cup liquid castile soap
- 1/4 cup brewed chamomile tea, cooled
- 1 tablespoon honey (optional, for added moisture)
- 10 drops lavender essential oil (for scent and additional calming properties)
- Glass bottle with pump dispenser

Instructions

1. Brew a strong cup of chamomile tea and allow it to cool to room temperature.
2. In a mixing bowl, combine the cold-pressed castor oil and liquid castile soap. Stir gently to mix.
3. Add the cooled chamomile tea to the oil and soap mixture. If using, incorporate the honey for extra moisturizing benefits.
4. Add the lavender essential oil to the mixture for a calming scent and additional skin-soothing effects.
5. Stir all the ingredients until well combined.
6. Using a funnel, carefully pour the body wash into a glass bottle with a pump dispenser for easy use in the shower or bath.
7. To use, pump a small amount onto a washcloth or directly onto your skin. Massage into a lather, then rinse thoroughly with water.

Variations

- For extra skin soothing, add a tablespoon of aloe vera gel to the mixture.

- If you prefer a different scent, substitute lavender essential oil with another skin-friendly essential oil like rose or geranium.

Storage tips
Store the body wash in a cool, dry place, away from direct sunlight. The glass bottle will help preserve the integrity of the essential oils and other natural ingredients. Use within 6 months for best quality.

Tips for allergens
If you have allergies to chamomile or lavender, you can omit these ingredients or substitute them with other skin-friendly ingredients that suit your needs. Always perform a patch test on a small area of your skin before using the body wash extensively, especially if you have sensitive skin or are prone to allergies.

Castor Oil and Peppermint Cooling Gel

Beneficial effects
The Castor Oil and Peppermint Cooling Gel offers a refreshing and soothing remedy for tired, achy muscles and skin irritation. The combination of castor oil's anti-inflammatory properties with peppermint's cooling effect provides immediate relief from discomfort, reduces redness and swelling, and promotes a sense of well-being. This gel is also excellent for post-sun care, helping to calm sunburned skin.

Ingredients
- 1/4 cup cold-pressed castor oil
- 1/4 cup aloe vera gel
- 10 drops peppermint essential oil
- 2 tablespoons witch hazel

Instructions
1. In a clean bowl, mix the aloe vera gel and witch hazel until well combined.
2. Slowly add the cold-pressed castor oil to the mixture, stirring continuously to ensure it blends smoothly with the aloe vera gel and witch hazel.
3. Add the peppermint essential oil to the mixture and stir thoroughly. The peppermint oil not only adds a cooling sensation but also enhances the anti-inflammatory benefits of the gel.
4. Transfer the gel into a clean, airtight container for storage.
5. To use, apply a small amount of the cooling gel to the affected area, gently massaging in circular motions. Reapply as needed for relief.

Variations
- For extra cooling effects, store the gel in the refrigerator before application.
- If you have sensitive skin, reduce the amount of peppermint essential oil to 5 drops to lessen the intensity of the cooling sensation.
- For an additional soothing effect, add 5 drops of lavender essential oil to the mixture.

Storage tips

Keep the Castor Oil and Peppermint Cooling Gel in an airtight container in the refrigerator. The cool environment will enhance the refreshing effect of the gel and help preserve its potency. Use within 1 month for best results.

Tips for allergens

If you are allergic to peppermint or any other ingredient listed, you can substitute peppermint essential oil with eucalyptus essential oil, which also provides a cooling effect but may be less irritating for some individuals. Always perform a patch test on a small area of your skin before using the gel extensively, especially if you have sensitive skin or are prone to allergies.

Castor Oil and Rose Water Body Mist

Beneficial effects

The Castor Oil and Rose Water Body Mist offers a refreshing and hydrating experience, ideal for soothing and revitalizing the skin. Castor oil, known for its anti-inflammatory and moisturizing properties, works in tandem with rose water, celebrated for its ability to tone, balance, and cool the skin. This mist is perfect for calming irritated or sun-exposed skin, setting makeup, or simply providing a moisture boost throughout the day. Its natural ingredients make it suitable for all skin types, promoting a balanced and radiant complexion.

Ingredients

- 1/4 cup distilled water
- 2 tablespoons cold-pressed castor oil
- 1/4 cup pure rose water
- 5 drops of lavender essential oil (optional for additional soothing effects)
- Small spray bottle

Instructions

1. In a clean bowl, mix the distilled water and cold-pressed castor oil thoroughly. The mixture may initially separate, so whisk vigorously to create a more cohesive blend.
2. Add the rose water to the oil and water mixture, continuing to whisk until all ingredients are well combined.
3. If using, incorporate the lavender essential oil for its calming properties and gentle fragrance. Stir well.
4. Using a funnel, carefully pour the mixture into the small spray bottle.
5. To use, shake the bottle well before each application to ensure the oil is mixed. Hold the bottle about six inches away from your face or body and lightly mist the skin. Allow to air dry or gently pat the skin with a clean cloth.
6. Apply as needed throughout the day for a refreshing and hydrating boost.

Variations
- For a cooling effect, especially in hot weather or after sun exposure, store the mist in the refrigerator before use.
- To target specific skin concerns, such as increased hydration or anti-aging, add a few drops of hyaluronic acid or rosehip seed oil to the mixture.

Storage tips
Store your body mist in the refrigerator to maintain freshness and enhance the cooling effect upon application. Use within 1-2 weeks for the best quality and efficacy.

Tips for allergens
If you are sensitive to lavender or any essential oils, you can omit them from the recipe. Always perform a patch test on a small area of your skin before using the mist extensively, especially if incorporating new ingredients into your skincare routine.

Castor Oil and Vitamin E Body Oil

Beneficial effects
The Castor Oil and Vitamin E Body Oil is a deeply nourishing and hydrating treatment designed to improve skin elasticity, reduce the appearance of scars and stretch marks, and provide an overall moisturizing effect. Castor oil, known for its anti-inflammatory and healing properties, works in synergy with Vitamin E, a potent antioxidant that helps to protect the skin from environmental stressors and UV damage. This combination not only moisturizes the skin but also aids in healing and rejuvenating, leaving the skin soft, supple, and radiant.

Ingredients
- 1/2 cup cold-pressed castor oil
- 1/4 cup Vitamin E oil
- 10 drops of lavender essential oil (optional for a calming scent and additional skin benefits)

Instructions
1. In a clean glass bowl, combine the cold-pressed castor oil with Vitamin E oil. Mix thoroughly to ensure the oils are well blended.
2. If using, add the lavender essential oil to the mixture and stir again to distribute the scent and its skin-soothing properties evenly throughout the oil.
3. Transfer the oil blend into a dark glass bottle with a pump or dropper for easy application.
4. To use, apply a small amount of the body oil to damp skin after showering. Gently massage in circular motions until fully absorbed. Focus on areas prone to dryness or where skin is stretched and scarred.
5. For best results, use daily to maintain skin hydration and elasticity.

Variations

- For added moisture, include a few drops of almond oil, which is rich in Vitamin A and E, to further nourish and soften the skin.
- If you have sensitive skin, you can substitute lavender essential oil with chamomile essential oil for its gentle and soothing properties.

Storage tips

Store the body oil in a cool, dark place to preserve the integrity of the oils and prevent oxidation. The dark glass bottle will help protect the oil from light, extending its shelf life. Ensure the bottle is tightly sealed after each use. The body oil should remain effective for up to 6 months when stored properly.

Tips for allergens

If you are sensitive to lavender or any other essential oils, you can omit them from the recipe. Always perform a patch test on a small area of your skin before using the body oil extensively, especially if you have sensitive skin or are prone to allergies.

Castor Oil and Green Tea Body Cream

Beneficial effects

The Castor Oil and Green Tea Body Cream offers a unique combination of deep moisturization from castor oil and the antioxidant benefits of green tea. This cream is designed to hydrate the skin, improve its elasticity, and protect against environmental damage. Castor oil's rich fatty acid content nourishes the skin deeply, while green tea, loaded with antioxidants, helps to repair and rejuvenate skin cells, reducing signs of aging and giving the skin a healthy glow.

Ingredients

- 1/4 cup cold-pressed castor oil
- 1/4 cup coconut oil
- 2 tablespoons beeswax
- 1/2 cup brewed green tea (cooled)
- 10 drops of vitamin E oil
- 5 drops of lavender essential oil (optional for scent and additional skin benefits)

Instructions

1. In a double boiler, melt the beeswax and coconut oil together until fully liquid.
2. Remove from heat and allow the mixture to cool slightly.
3. Slowly stir in the cold-pressed castor oil, ensuring it's well integrated.
4. Gradually add the brewed green tea to the mixture, stirring continuously. The mixture should start to thicken as you stir.
5. Mix in the vitamin E oil and, if using, the lavender essential oil, until the mixture is homogeneous.
6. Pour the cream into a clean, dry jar and allow it to cool and solidify at room temperature.
7. Once solidified, seal the jar. Your body cream is now ready for use.

Variations

- For added anti-inflammatory properties, include a few drops of chamomile essential oil in the mixture.
- If you prefer a vegan option, substitute beeswax with an equal amount of candelilla wax.

Storage tips

Store your body cream in a cool, dry place, away from direct sunlight. If stored properly, the cream should remain effective for up to 3 months. Ensure the jar is tightly sealed to maintain the cream's potency.

Tips for allergens

If you have a sensitivity to coconut oil, you can substitute it with jojoba oil, which is also excellent for skin health and less likely to cause irritation. Always perform a patch test on a small area of your skin before applying the cream extensively, especially if you have sensitive skin or are prone to allergies.

Oral Health and Eye Care Remedies

Castor Oil and Clove Oil Mouthwash

Beneficial effects
The Castor Oil and Clove Oil Mouthwash is designed to enhance oral health by leveraging the antibacterial properties of both castor oil and clove oil. This mouthwash can help in reducing gum inflammation, alleviating toothache, and combating bad breath. Castor oil, with its antimicrobial qualities, aids in cleansing the mouth, while clove oil, known for its eugenol content, provides a natural analgesic effect that can soothe tooth and gum pain.

Ingredients
- 2 tablespoons of cold-pressed castor oil
- 5 drops of clove essential oil
- 1 cup of distilled water
- 1 teaspoon of sea salt (optional, for added antimicrobial properties)

Instructions
1. In a clean glass jar, combine the distilled water and cold-pressed castor oil. Shake well to mix.
2. Add the clove essential oil to the jar. If using, also add the sea salt. Close the jar and shake vigorously to ensure all ingredients are thoroughly mixed.
3. To use, swish a small amount of the mouthwash in your mouth for 1-2 minutes, then spit it out. Do not swallow.
4. Use this mouthwash twice daily after brushing your teeth, in the morning and before bed, for best results.

Variations
- For a refreshing flavor and additional antibacterial benefits, add 2 drops of peppermint essential oil to the mixture.
- If you have sensitive gums, you can reduce the amount of clove oil to 2-3 drops to lessen the intensity.

Storage tips
Store the mouthwash in a cool, dark place. The glass jar should be tightly sealed to preserve the potency of the essential oils. Use within 1 month for optimal freshness and efficacy.

Tips for allergens
If you are allergic to clove oil, you can substitute it with tea tree oil, which also has potent antimicrobial properties suitable for oral care. Always perform a patch test on your skin before using the mouthwash if you're incorporating essential oils for the first time, to ensure there is no adverse reaction.

Castor Oil and Peppermint Toothpaste

Beneficial effects
The Castor Oil and Peppermint Toothpaste is a natural, fluoride-free alternative designed to clean teeth, freshen breath, and promote oral health. Castor oil's antibacterial properties help fight oral bacteria, while peppermint oil provides a refreshing taste and naturally whitens teeth. Together, they create a powerful combination that not only cleans but also soothes gums and reduces inflammation.

Ingredients
- 2 tablespoons of cold-pressed castor oil
- 2 tablespoons of baking soda
- 2 tablespoons of coconut oil
- 10-15 drops of peppermint essential oil
- 1 teaspoon of xylitol (optional, for sweetness)

Instructions
1. In a small bowl, mix the cold-pressed castor oil and coconut oil until well combined.
2. Gradually add the baking soda to the oil mixture, stirring continuously until a paste forms.
3. Add the peppermint essential oil to the paste, adjusting the amount based on your preference for flavor intensity.
4. If desired, incorporate the xylitol into the mixture for added sweetness.
5. Transfer the toothpaste into a small, airtight container for storage.

Variations
- For added whitening properties, include a teaspoon of activated charcoal powder to the mixture.
- If you prefer a different flavor, substitute peppermint essential oil with cinnamon or spearmint essential oil.

Storage tips
Store the toothpaste in a cool, dry place. Ensure the container is tightly sealed to maintain freshness. The toothpaste should remain effective for up to 3 months.

Tips for allergens
If you're sensitive to coconut oil, you can substitute it with additional castor oil or olive oil. Always perform a patch test on a small area inside your mouth before using the toothpaste extensively, especially if you're incorporating new ingredients into your oral care routine.

Castor Oil and Baking Soda Teeth Whitener

Beneficial effects
The Castor Oil and Baking Soda Teeth Whitener offers a natural, effective solution for removing stains and whitening teeth. Castor oil, known for its antibacterial properties, helps in reducing plaque buildup and promoting oral health. Baking soda, on the other hand, acts as a gentle abrasive that effectively removes

surface stains from the teeth, restoring their natural whiteness. This combination not only brightens the teeth but also contributes to a healthier oral environment.

Ingredients
-   2 tablespoons of cold-pressed castor oil
-   2 tablespoons of baking soda
-   2-3 drops of peppermint essential oil (optional for fresh breath)

Instructions
1. In a small bowl, mix the castor oil and baking soda until you achieve a paste-like consistency.
2. If using, add the peppermint essential oil to the mixture and stir well. This step is optional but recommended for those who prefer a minty freshness.
3. Apply a small amount of the paste to your toothbrush and brush your teeth gently for 2 minutes, focusing on areas with more noticeable stains.
4. Rinse your mouth thoroughly with water after brushing.
5. Use this whitening treatment 2-3 times a week in place of your regular toothpaste.

Variations
-   For added antibacterial properties, you can include a drop of tea tree essential oil into the mixture.
-   If you have sensitive teeth, reduce the amount of baking soda to 1 tablespoon to minimize abrasiveness.

Storage tips
Prepare the mixture fresh each time to ensure the best results and to maintain the potency of the essential oils if used. It's not recommended to store any leftovers due to the potential for the baking soda to react with moisture in the air.

Tips for allergens
If you are sensitive to peppermint or tea tree oil, you can omit these from the recipe. Always perform a patch test on the inside of your wrist before using the mixture to ensure there is no adverse reaction, especially when incorporating essential oils for the first time.

Castor Oil and Turmeric Gum Treatment

Beneficial effects
The Castor Oil and Turmeric Gum Treatment is an effective natural remedy designed to improve oral health, reduce gum inflammation, and alleviate pain. Castor oil's antibacterial properties help fight oral pathogens, while turmeric's curcumin content offers powerful anti-inflammatory and analgesic benefits. Together, they form a potent combination that can help in treating gum disease, soothing sore gums, and maintaining overall oral hygiene.

Ingredients
-   2 tablespoons of cold-pressed castor oil

- 1 teaspoon of turmeric powder
- 1/2 teaspoon of salt (optional, for its antiseptic properties)
- Warm water (for rinsing)

Instructions

1. In a small bowl, mix the cold-pressed castor oil and turmeric powder until you achieve a paste-like consistency.
2. If using, add the salt to the mixture and blend well. The salt acts as an additional antiseptic agent to further support oral health.
3. Apply a small amount of the paste directly onto the gums using a clean fingertip or a soft toothbrush. Gently massage the gums with the paste, covering all areas, especially those that are sore or inflamed.
4. Leave the paste on your gums for 5 to 10 minutes to allow the active ingredients to penetrate and exert their effects.
5. Rinse your mouth thoroughly with warm water to remove the paste. Ensure all residue is washed away.
6. Repeat this treatment once daily, preferably before bedtime, to maximize healing and anti-inflammatory benefits overnight.

Variations

- For enhanced antimicrobial effects, add 2 drops of peppermint essential oil to the mixture. Peppermint will also leave a refreshing aftertaste and can help in neutralizing bad breath.
- If the paste's consistency is too thick, a small amount of coconut oil can be added to make the application smoother and add additional antimicrobial properties.

Storage tips

Prepare this treatment fresh each time to ensure the potency of turmeric and castor oil. It's best not to store any prepared mixture as the turmeric may lose its efficacy over time when mixed and not stored properly.

Tips for allergens

If you are allergic to turmeric or castor oil, it's crucial to perform a patch test before applying the mixture to your gums. In case of a reaction, discontinue use immediately. For individuals with sensitivity to peppermint oil, omit this ingredient or replace it with a milder essential oil like chamomile, which also possesses soothing properties.

Castor Oil and Coconut Oil, Oil Pulling Solution

Beneficial effects

The Castor Oil and Coconut Oil Oil Pulling Solution is designed to improve oral health by removing bacteria, reducing plaque, and promoting healthy gums. This ancient Ayurvedic practice not only detoxifies the mouth but also contributes to overall health by reducing systemic inflammation and improving bad breath.

Ingredients
- 1 tablespoon of cold-pressed castor oil
- 1 tablespoon of virgin coconut oil

Instructions
1. In a small bowl, mix together the cold-pressed castor oil and virgin coconut oil until they are well combined.
2. Take a tablespoon of the mixture into your mouth first thing in the morning before you eat or drink anything.
3. Swish the oil around your mouth, pulling it through your teeth and around your gums for 15-20 minutes. It's important not to swallow the oil as it contains toxins and bacteria pulled from your gums.
4. After 15-20 minutes, spit the oil into a trash can to avoid clogging your sink.
5. Rinse your mouth well with warm water, then proceed with your usual oral hygiene routine, brushing and flossing as normal.

Variations
- For added antimicrobial properties, you can add 2 drops of tea tree essential oil to the mixture.
- If you prefer a minty freshness, include 1-2 drops of peppermint essential oil to enhance the oil pulling experience and freshen breath.

Storage tips
Prepare the mixture fresh each morning to ensure the best quality and effectiveness. If you prefer to prepare in advance, store the oil mixture in a sealed glass jar in a cool, dark place for up to a week.

Tips for allergens
If you are allergic to coconut oil, the oil pulling solution can be made with castor oil alone, or you can substitute coconut oil with sesame oil, which is also traditionally used for oil pulling and has similar antibacterial properties. Always ensure you are not allergic to any essential oils used in the variations by performing a patch test on your skin before adding them to your oil pulling routine.

Castor Oil and Aloe Vera Eye Drops

Beneficial effects
Castor Oil and Aloe Vera Eye Drops are designed to soothe dry, irritated eyes, providing moisture and relief with natural anti-inflammatory and hydrating properties. Castor oil helps to stabilize the tear film and reduce evaporation, while aloe vera offers gentle soothing and healing benefits, making this remedy ideal for those suffering from dry eye syndrome, irritation from environmental factors, or discomfort from prolonged screen use.

Ingredients
- 2 tablespoons of cold-pressed castor oil, hexane-free
- 1 tablespoon of pure aloe vera gel, ensure it's preservative-free and suitable for internal use

- 1/4 cup of distilled water, boiled and cooled to ensure sterility

Instructions

1. Start by sterilizing a small glass dropper bottle and all utensils with boiling water to eliminate any potential contaminants. Allow them to dry completely before use.
2. In a sterilized bowl, mix the aloe vera gel with the distilled water until fully combined.
3. Add the cold-pressed castor oil to the aloe mixture, stirring gently to ensure a homogeneous blend.
4. Using a sterilized funnel, carefully transfer the mixture into the sterilized glass dropper bottle.
5. To use, apply 1-2 drops in each eye before bedtime. Blink several times to distribute the drops evenly.
6. Store the eye drops in the refrigerator to preserve freshness. Use within one week to ensure sterility and effectiveness.

Variations

- For additional soothing effects, especially after exposure to wind or sun, you can add a drop of vitamin E oil to the mixture. Vitamin E has antioxidant properties that can help protect and repair the skin around the eyes.
- If you experience mild eye irritation or allergies, adding a pinch of turmeric powder can provide additional anti-inflammatory benefits. Ensure it's completely dissolved and strain the mixture through a fine cloth to remove any particles before use.

Storage tips

Keep the eye drops refrigerated and tightly sealed when not in use. The cool temperature helps maintain the efficacy of the ingredients and provides an additional soothing effect upon application. Discard any unused drops after one week to avoid the risk of contamination.

Tips for allergens

If you have sensitivity to aloe vera or castor oil, it's crucial to perform a patch test on a small area of your arm before applying the drops to your eyes. Should any irritation occur, discontinue use immediately. For those allergic to aloe vera, substituting it with saline solution can offer a simple, yet effective alternative for mixing with the castor oil.

Castor Oil and Chamomile Eye Compress

Beneficial effects

The Castor Oil and Chamomile Eye Compress offers a soothing, natural remedy for reducing eye puffiness, irritation, and dark circles. Castor oil's anti-inflammatory properties help soothe swollen eyelids and under-eye areas, while chamomile's calming effects reduce redness and provide a relaxing experience. Together, they create a potent treatment that not only alleviates discomfort but also rejuvenates the delicate skin around the eyes, promoting a refreshed and bright appearance.

Ingredients

- 2 tablespoons of cold-pressed castor oil

- 1 chamomile tea bag or 1 tablespoon of dried chamomile flowers
- 1/2 cup of boiling water
- 2 clean, soft cloths or cotton pads

Instructions

1. Steep the chamomile tea bag or dried chamomile flowers in the boiling water for about 10 minutes to make a strong chamomile tea. Allow the tea to cool to a comfortable, warm temperature.
2. While the tea is cooling, soak the clean cloths or cotton pads in cold-pressed castor oil. Ensure they are fully saturated but not dripping.
3. Remove the chamomile tea bag or strain the flowers from the water. Soak the castor oil-saturated cloths or cotton pads in the warm chamomile tea, allowing them to absorb the tea.
4. Gently squeeze out any excess liquid from the cloths or cotton pads to prevent dripping.
5. Lie down and place the soaked cloths or cotton pads over your closed eyelids. Relax and leave the compress on for 15-20 minutes.
6. Remove the compress and gently pat the eye area dry with a clean towel. Follow up with a light moisturizer if desired.

Variations

- For additional cooling effects, which can further reduce puffiness, chill the chamomile tea in the refrigerator before soaking the cloths or cotton pads.
- If chamomile is not available, green tea can be used as an alternative due to its antioxidant properties and soothing effects on the skin.

Storage tips

Prepare the chamomile tea fresh for each use to ensure the best results. The cold-pressed castor oil should be stored in a cool, dark place to maintain its potency. Any unused castor oil can be kept for future applications.

Tips for allergens

If you have allergies to chamomile, opting for green tea as suggested in the variations can provide a similar soothing effect without the allergen. Always perform a patch test on the inside of your wrist with both the castor oil and the chosen tea to ensure there is no adverse reaction before applying the compress to your eye area.

Castor Oil and Green Tea Eye Serum

Beneficial effects

The Castor Oil and Green Tea Eye Serum is designed to rejuvenate and brighten the delicate skin around the eyes. Castor oil, rich in fatty acids, deeply moisturizes and reduces the appearance of fine lines, while green tea, loaded with antioxidants, helps to diminish dark circles and puffiness. This serum offers a natural, gentle solution for enhancing eye area health, providing a refreshed and youthful appearance.

Ingredients
- 2 tablespoons of cold-pressed castor oil
- 1 tablespoon of green tea extract
- 1 teaspoon of vitamin E oil
- 5 drops of chamomile essential oil

Instructions
1. Begin by mixing the cold-pressed castor oil with the green tea extract in a small bowl. Ensure the two are well combined to form the base of your serum.
2. Add the vitamin E oil to the mixture. Vitamin E acts as a natural preservative and adds additional antioxidant properties to the serum.
3. Incorporate the chamomile essential oil into the serum. Chamomile provides calming and soothing benefits, ideal for the sensitive skin around the eyes.
4. Once all the ingredients are thoroughly mixed, transfer the serum to a clean, dark glass dropper bottle to protect the oils from light degradation.
5. To use, gently apply a few drops of the serum around the eye area, being careful to avoid direct contact with the eyes. For best results, use the serum nightly before bed.

Variations
- For an added cooling effect, which can help reduce puffiness more effectively, store the serum in the refrigerator.
- If chamomile essential oil is not available or if you're looking for a different scent, lavender essential oil can be used as an alternative. It also offers soothing properties beneficial for the skin.

Storage tips
Keep the eye serum in a cool, dark place, ideally in the refrigerator, to maintain its freshness and efficacy. When stored properly, the serum should remain effective for up to 6 months.

Tips for allergens
If you have sensitive skin or are allergic to any of the essential oils, you can omit them from the recipe. Always perform a patch test on the inside of your wrist before applying the serum to your face to ensure there is no adverse reaction.

Castor Oil and Rose Water Eye Mist

Beneficial effects
The Castor Oil and Rose Water Eye Mist is designed to refresh, hydrate, and soothe the delicate skin around the eyes. Castor oil, with its anti-inflammatory and moisturizing properties, helps to reduce puffiness and under-eye bags, while rose water offers a calming effect, reducing redness and irritation. This gentle mist can also help to tighten the skin around the eyes, providing a more youthful appearance.

Ingredients
- 2 tablespoons of cold-pressed castor oil

- 1/2 cup of pure rose water
- 1/4 cup of distilled water
- 5 drops of vitamin E oil (optional for added antioxidant benefits)
- Small spray bottle

Instructions

1. In a clean bowl, mix the cold-pressed castor oil with distilled water thoroughly.
2. Add the rose water to the oil and water mixture, continuing to mix until well combined.
3. If using, incorporate the vitamin E oil into the mixture for its skin-nourishing properties.
4. Using a funnel, carefully pour the mixture into the small spray bottle.
5. To use, gently shake the bottle before each application to ensure the oils are well mixed. Close your eyes and lightly mist around the eye area, keeping the bottle a few inches away from your face. Allow the mist to air dry or gently pat the area with a clean cloth.
6. Apply in the morning to refresh and hydrate your skin or throughout the day as needed for a soothing boost.

Variations

- For additional soothing benefits, especially for sensitive skin, add 2 drops of chamomile essential oil to the mixture.
- To enhance the cooling effect, store the eye mist in the refrigerator before use.

Storage tips

Keep the eye mist in a cool, dark place when not in use. If stored in the refrigerator, the mist can provide an extra cooling sensation upon application and can last for up to 2 weeks.

Tips for allergens

If you are sensitive to any of the ingredients, particularly essential oils, you can omit them from the recipe. Always perform a patch test on the inside of your wrist before using the mist around your eyes, especially if you have sensitive skin or are prone to allergies.

Castor Oil and Vitamin E Eye Cream

Beneficial effects

The Castor Oil and Vitamin E Eye Cream is specifically formulated to hydrate and rejuvenate the delicate skin around the eyes. This cream combines the anti-inflammatory and moisturizing properties of castor oil with the antioxidant benefits of Vitamin E, helping to reduce the appearance of fine lines, dark circles, and puffiness. Regular use can promote a more youthful, radiant look around the eyes by deeply nourishing the skin, protecting it from environmental stressors, and improving its overall texture.

Ingredients

- 2 tablespoons of cold-pressed castor oil
- 1 tablespoon of Vitamin E oil
- 1 tablespoon of aloe vera gel

- 5 drops of lavender essential oil (optional for additional soothing effects and a pleasant scent)
- Small glass jar for storage

Instructions

1. In a clean bowl, mix the cold-pressed castor oil and Vitamin E oil until well combined.
2. Add the aloe vera gel to the oil mixture and stir thoroughly to achieve a smooth, consistent cream.
3. If using, incorporate the lavender essential oil into the cream for its calming properties and gentle fragrance.
4. Carefully transfer the eye cream into a small glass jar.
5. To apply, gently dab a small amount of the cream around the eyes with your ring finger, avoiding direct contact with the eyes. Use every night before bed for best results.

Variations

- For extra cooling and de-puffing benefits, store the eye cream in the refrigerator. The cool temperature will enhance the soothing effect when applied.
- If sensitive to lavender, substitute with chamomile essential oil, which is also known for its soothing and anti-inflammatory properties.

Storage tips

Keep the eye cream in a cool, dark place, ideally in the refrigerator, to maintain its freshness and potency. Ensure the jar is tightly sealed to prevent air exposure. The cream should be used within 6 months for optimal benefits.

Tips for allergens

For those with sensitivities to essential oils, the lavender essential oil can be omitted without affecting the cream's effectiveness. Always perform a patch test on a small area of your forearm before applying near the eyes, especially if you have sensitive skin or are prone to allergies.

Digestive Health Recipes

Castor Oil and Ginger Digestive Tonic

Beneficial effects
The Castor Oil and Ginger Digestive Tonic is a natural remedy designed to aid digestion, soothe stomach discomfort, and reduce inflammation. Castor oil's anti-inflammatory properties help to calm the digestive tract, while ginger is renowned for its ability to alleviate nausea, bloating, and indigestion. Together, they create a potent tonic that can promote a healthy digestive system, ease discomfort, and support overall gut health.

Ingredients
- 2 tablespoons of cold-pressed castor oil
- 1 tablespoon of fresh ginger juice
- 1 cup of warm water
- 1 teaspoon of honey (optional, for taste)

Instructions
1. Extract the juice from fresh ginger using a juicer or by grating the ginger and pressing it through a fine mesh sieve.
2. Warm the water to a comfortable drinking temperature. Do not boil, as extreme heat can degrade the beneficial properties of the castor oil.
3. In a mug, combine the warm water, cold-pressed castor oil, and fresh ginger juice. Stir well to ensure the ingredients are fully mixed.
4. If desired, add a teaspoon of honey to the mixture and stir until dissolved. This step is optional but can improve the taste of the tonic.
5. Drink the tonic first thing in the morning on an empty stomach to maximize its digestive benefits.

Variations
- For added digestive support, include a pinch of ground cinnamon or turmeric to the tonic. Both spices have anti-inflammatory properties and can enhance the tonic's effectiveness.
- If you find the taste of castor oil too strong, reduce the amount to 1 tablespoon and gradually increase it as you become accustomed to the flavor.

Storage tips
Prepare this tonic fresh each morning to ensure the potency of the ingredients. It's best not to store the mixture, as the fresh ginger juice and castor oil are most effective when consumed immediately after preparation.

Tips for allergens
If you are allergic to honey, you can substitute it with maple syrup or simply omit the sweetener altogether. Always ensure that you are not allergic to any of the ingredients by performing a patch test or consulting with a healthcare provider before incorporating this tonic into your routine.

Castor Oil and Peppermint Digestive Aid

Beneficial effects

The Castor Oil and Peppermint Digestive Aid is a natural remedy designed to soothe digestive discomfort, reduce bloating, and promote healthy digestion. Castor oil, with its anti-inflammatory properties, assists in calming the digestive tract, while peppermint oil is known for its ability to relieve indigestion, gas, and bloating. This combination not only aids in digestion but also provides a refreshing, cooling sensation that can help ease stomach discomfort.

Ingredients

- 2 tablespoons of cold-pressed castor oil
- 3-4 drops of peppermint essential oil
- 1 cup of warm water

Instructions

1. Add the cold-pressed castor oil to the cup of warm water.
2. Incorporate 3-4 drops of peppermint essential oil into the mixture.
3. Stir the mixture thoroughly until both oils are well dispersed in the water.
4. Drink this mixture first thing in the morning on an empty stomach or 30 minutes before meals to aid digestion.

Variations

- For those who find the taste of castor oil too strong, mixing the oils with a small amount of organic honey can help mask the flavor.
- If experiencing severe bloating, increasing the peppermint essential oil to 5 drops may provide additional relief.

Storage tips

Prepare this digestive aid fresh each time to ensure the effectiveness of the essential oils and castor oil. It is not recommended to store any premixed solution as the potency of the essential oils may diminish over time.

Tips for allergens

If you are sensitive to peppermint, you can substitute it with ginger essential oil, which also offers digestive benefits. Always perform a patch test on your skin before consuming essential oils, especially if you have a history of allergies or sensitive skin.

Castor Oil and Fennel Seed Stomach Soother

Beneficial effects

The Castor Oil and Fennel Seed Stomach Soother is designed to alleviate digestive discomfort, reduce bloating, and promote a healthy digestive system. Castor oil's anti-inflammatory properties help soothe irritated digestive tracts, while fennel seeds are known for their ability to relieve gas, bloating, and stomach cramps. This natural remedy supports overall digestive health and provides relief from discomfort.

Ingredients
- 2 tablespoons of cold-pressed castor oil
- 1 teaspoon of crushed fennel seeds
- 1 cup of boiling water

Instructions
1. Place the crushed fennel seeds in a cup or mug.
2. Pour the boiling water over the fennel seeds and let them steep for 10 minutes.
3. Strain the fennel seeds from the water and allow the fennel tea to cool to a comfortable temperature.
4. Stir in the cold-pressed castor oil into the cooled fennel tea until well combined.
5. Drink the mixture slowly. For best results, consume this stomach soother on an empty stomach in the morning or before meals.

Variations
- For added flavor and digestive benefits, include a teaspoon of honey or a slice of ginger while steeping the fennel seeds.
- If you find the taste of castor oil too strong, you can reduce the amount to 1 tablespoon and gradually increase it as you become accustomed to the flavor.

Storage tips
Prepare the Castor Oil and Fennel Seed Stomach Soother fresh for each use to ensure maximum potency and effectiveness. It is not recommended to store any leftovers due to the quick degradation of the active properties when mixed.

Tips for allergens
If you are allergic to fennel seeds, you can substitute them with peppermint leaves, which also offer digestive benefits and can help soothe stomach discomfort. Always ensure that you are not allergic to any of the ingredients by performing a patch test or consulting with a healthcare provider before use.

Castor Oil and Lemon Digestive Cleanse

Beneficial effects
The Castor Oil and Lemon Digestive Cleanse is designed to support digestive health by leveraging the detoxifying properties of lemon and the laxative effects of castor oil. This combination stimulates the digestive system, helps in the removal of toxins, and encourages a healthy bowel movement. Regular use can lead to improved gut health, reduced bloating, and a more efficient digestive process.

Ingredients
- 1 tablespoon of cold-pressed, hexane-free castor oil
- Juice of 1/2 organic lemon

- 1 cup of warm water

Instructions
1. Squeeze the juice of half a lemon into a cup of warm water. Ensure the water is not too hot to preserve the nutritional properties of the lemon juice.
2. Add 1 tablespoon of cold-pressed, hexane-free castor oil to the lemon water.
3. Stir the mixture well until the castor oil is fully dispersed.
4. Drink this mixture on an empty stomach in the morning, ideally as soon as you wake up.
5. Wait at least 30 minutes before eating breakfast to allow your body to absorb the drink's benefits.

Variations
- For added flavor and detoxifying properties, you can include a teaspoon of organic honey or a pinch of cayenne pepper.
- If you find the taste of castor oil too strong, mixing it with a small amount of orange juice instead of water can help mask the flavor.

Storage tips
Store your castor oil in a cool, dark place to maintain its freshness and efficacy. The lemon should be stored in the refrigerator and used within a week for the best flavor and health benefits.

Tips for allergens
Individuals with sensitivity to citrus or castor oil should start with a smaller dose to ensure no adverse reactions occur. If you experience any discomfort or allergic reactions, discontinue use immediately and consult a healthcare provider.

Castor Oil and Chamomile Digestive Tea

Beneficial effects
The Castor Oil and Chamomile Digestive Tea is a soothing blend designed to alleviate digestive discomfort, reduce inflammation, and promote relaxation. Castor oil, with its anti-inflammatory properties, aids in soothing the digestive tract, while chamomile is renowned for its calming effects on the stomach, helping to ease cramps, reduce bloating, and improve overall digestion.

Ingredients
- 1 tablespoon of cold-pressed castor oil
- 1 chamomile tea bag or 1 tablespoon of dried chamomile flowers
- 1 cup of boiling water
- Honey or lemon to taste (optional)

Instructions
1. Place the chamomile tea bag or dried chamomile flowers in a cup.
2. Pour 1 cup of boiling water over the chamomile and allow it to steep for 5-10 minutes.
3. Remove the tea bag or strain the tea to remove the flowers.

4. Stir in 1 tablespoon of cold-pressed castor oil into the warm chamomile tea until well combined.

5. If desired, add honey or lemon to taste for additional flavor.

6. Drink the tea slowly, preferably before bedtime, to allow the soothing properties to work overnight.

Variations

- For additional digestive benefits, add a pinch of ginger powder to the tea while steeping. Ginger enhances the anti-inflammatory and soothing effects.

- If you prefer a cooler beverage, allow the tea to cool to room temperature before adding the castor oil, then refrigerate for a refreshing cold drink.

Storage tips

It's best to prepare this tea fresh each time to ensure the potency of the ingredients. However, the chamomile tea (without castor oil) can be brewed in larger quantities and stored in the refrigerator for up to 2 days. Add castor oil to individual servings as needed.

Tips for allergens

If you have allergies to chamomile, consider substituting it with peppermint or fennel tea, both of which also offer digestive benefits. Always ensure that the castor oil is cold-pressed and hexane-free to avoid potential irritants.

Castor Oil and Apple Cider Vinegar Digestive Elixir

Beneficial effects

The Castor Oil and Apple Cider Vinegar Digestive Elixir is a natural remedy designed to improve digestive health, balance stomach acid levels, and support the body's detoxification processes. Castor oil's anti-inflammatory and antimicrobial properties help soothe the digestive tract, while apple cider vinegar aids in digestion and nutrient absorption, making this elixir particularly beneficial for those experiencing bloating, indigestion, or irregular bowel movements.

Ingredients

- 1 tablespoon of cold-pressed castor oil
- 2 tablespoons of organic apple cider vinegar
- 1 cup of warm water
- 1 teaspoon of honey (optional, for taste)

Instructions

1. Measure 1 tablespoon of cold-pressed castor oil and pour it into a glass.

2. Add 2 tablespoons of organic apple cider vinegar to the glass.

3. Fill the glass with 1 cup of warm water to dilute the mixture, making it easier to consume.

4. If desired, add 1 teaspoon of honey to the mixture and stir well to improve the taste.

5. Drink the elixir first thing in the morning on an empty stomach to maximize its digestive health benefits.

Variations

- For added digestive support, include a pinch of ground ginger or cayenne pepper to the elixir. Both spices are known for their ability to stimulate digestion and improve circulation.
- If the taste of apple cider vinegar is too strong, increase the amount of honey to 2 teaspoons or substitute it with maple syrup for a different flavor profile.

Storage tips

Prepare the digestive elixir fresh each morning to ensure the best taste and potency of the ingredients. It is not recommended to store the mixture as the properties of castor oil and apple cider vinegar are most effective when fresh.

Tips for allergens

If you are allergic to honey, you can omit it from the recipe or substitute it with a small amount of stevia or agave syrup for sweetness. Always ensure that you are not allergic to any of the ingredients by performing a patch test or consulting with a healthcare provider before incorporating the elixir into your routine.

Castor Oil and Aloe Vera Digestive Gel

Beneficial effects

The Castor Oil and Aloe Vera Digestive Gel combines the soothing and anti-inflammatory properties of aloe vera with the detoxifying and cleansing benefits of castor oil to support digestive health. This gel can help soothe irritated digestive tracts, promote regularity, and aid in the natural detoxification process of the body. It's particularly beneficial for those experiencing constipation, bloating, or discomfort in the digestive system.

Ingredients

- 2 tablespoons of cold-pressed castor oil
- 1/2 cup of pure aloe vera gel
- 1 tablespoon of lemon juice (optional, for flavor and added digestive benefits)
- 1/2 cup of water

Instructions

1. In a blender, combine the aloe vera gel, cold-pressed castor oil, and water. Blend until the mixture reaches a smooth, gel-like consistency.
2. If using, add the lemon juice to the mixture and blend for an additional few seconds to incorporate.
3. Pour the digestive gel into a clean, airtight container.
4. To use, consume 1 tablespoon of the gel in the morning on an empty stomach. Wait at least 30 minutes before eating breakfast.

Variations

- For added digestive support, mix in 1 teaspoon of ground ginger or turmeric powder to the blend. Both spices are known for their anti-inflammatory and digestive health benefits.

- If the taste is too bland, add a tablespoon of honey to sweeten the gel naturally and provide additional soothing properties.

Storage tips
Store the digestive gel in the refrigerator in an airtight container to maintain freshness. Use within one week for optimal benefits.

Tips for allergens
If you are sensitive to aloe vera, start with a small dose to ensure it does not irritate your system. Always consult with a healthcare provider before incorporating new remedies into your health regimen, especially if you have existing health conditions or are taking medication.

Castor Oil and Turmeric Digestive Booster

Beneficial effects
The Castor Oil and Turmeric Digestive Booster is designed to support digestive health by leveraging the anti-inflammatory properties of turmeric and the laxative effects of castor oil. This combination aids in reducing digestive discomfort, enhancing bile flow, and facilitating the healing process of the digestive tract lining, making it beneficial for those suffering from bloating, gas, and irregular bowel movements.

Ingredients
- 1 tablespoon of cold-pressed castor oil
- 1/2 teaspoon of turmeric powder
- 1 cup of warm water
- Honey to taste (optional, for sweetness)

Instructions
1. Warm the water to a comfortable drinking temperature.
2. Add the turmeric powder to the warm water and stir until it is completely dissolved.
3. Incorporate the cold-pressed castor oil into the turmeric mixture and mix well.
4. If desired, add honey to taste for sweetness.
5. Drink this mixture on an empty stomach in the morning to maximize its digestive benefits.

Variations
- For an added boost, include a pinch of black pepper to the mixture. Piperine, found in black pepper, enhances the absorption of curcumin, the active compound in turmeric.
- Substitute warm water with warm almond milk for a creamier texture and additional health benefits.

Storage tips
Prepare this digestive booster fresh each morning to ensure the potency of the ingredients. It is not recommended to store any prepared mixture as the effectiveness may diminish over time.

Tips for allergens

If you are allergic to any of the ingredients listed, particularly honey, it can be omitted without significantly affecting the remedy's benefits. Always ensure you are not allergic to turmeric or castor oil by performing a patch test prior to ingestion, especially if you have a history of food sensitivities or allergies.

Castor Oil and Licorice Root Digestive Balm

Beneficial effects

The Castor Oil and Licorice Root Digestive Balm is a natural remedy crafted to soothe digestive discomfort, reduce inflammation in the gastrointestinal tract, and promote overall digestive health. Castor oil, with its anti-inflammatory properties, works to ease abdominal pain and discomfort, while licorice root, known for its soothing and healing effects on the digestive system, helps in treating issues like heartburn, indigestion, and stomach ulcers.

Ingredients
- 2 tablespoons of cold-pressed castor oil
- 1 tablespoon of licorice root powder
- 2 tablespoons of beeswax pellets
- 5 drops of peppermint essential oil (optional for additional digestive benefits and refreshing scent)
- Small glass jar for storage

Instructions
1. In a double boiler, melt the beeswax pellets over low heat until completely liquid.
2. Stir in the cold-pressed castor oil and licorice root powder into the melted beeswax. Mix thoroughly to ensure the ingredients are well combined.
3. Remove the mixture from heat and allow it to cool slightly.
4. If using, add the peppermint essential oil to the mixture and stir well. The peppermint oil can provide additional relief from digestive discomfort and improve the balm's scent.
5. Carefully pour the mixture into a small glass jar and allow it to cool and solidify at room temperature.
6. Once solidified, seal the jar. Your digestive balm is ready for use.

Variations
- For those sensitive to peppermint, ginger essential oil can be used as an alternative, offering warming digestive relief.
- If a softer balm is preferred, reduce the amount of beeswax to 1 tablespoon. This will make the balm easier to apply, especially in warmer climates.

Storage tips

Store the Castor Oil and Licorice Root Digestive Balm in a cool, dry place to maintain its consistency and potency. Ensure the jar is tightly sealed to prevent the balm from drying out. The balm should remain effective for up to 6 months when stored properly.

Tips for allergens

Individuals with sensitivities or allergies to licorice root should perform a patch test on a small area of the skin before applying the balm extensively. If an allergic reaction occurs, discontinue use immediately. For those allergic to beeswax, a plant-based wax like candelilla wax can be used as a suitable alternative.

Castor Oil and Cinnamon Digestive Support

Beneficial effects

The Castor Oil and Cinnamon Digestive Support is a natural remedy designed to aid digestion, soothe stomach discomfort, and reduce bloating. Castor oil acts as a stimulant laxative, providing relief from constipation, while cinnamon is known for its anti-inflammatory properties that can help alleviate digestive issues such as indigestion and gas. Together, they create a powerful blend that supports the digestive system, promoting overall gut health.

Ingredients

- 2 tablespoons of cold-pressed castor oil
- 1 teaspoon of ground cinnamon
- 1 cup of warm water
- Honey to taste (optional, for sweetness)

Instructions

1. Warm the water to a comfortable drinking temperature.
2. Add the ground cinnamon to the warm water and stir well to combine.
3. Incorporate the cold-pressed castor oil into the cinnamon water. Mix thoroughly until the oil is well dispersed.
4. If desired, add honey to taste for sweetness, and stir again to ensure all ingredients are evenly blended.
5. Drink the mixture on an empty stomach, preferably in the morning, to aid digestion throughout the day.

Variations

- For an added boost of digestive support, squeeze the juice of half a lemon into the mixture. Lemon can help detoxify the liver and promote bile production, aiding in digestion.
- If you prefer a cooler beverage, allow the mixture to cool to room temperature or add a few ice cubes before drinking.

Storage tips

It's best to prepare this digestive support drink fresh each time to ensure the potency of the ingredients and achieve the best results. However, if you need to prepare it in advance, store it in the refrigerator for no more than 24 hours to maintain freshness.

Tips for allergens

If you have a sensitivity to cinnamon, start with a smaller amount (1/2 teaspoon) and gradually increase to assess tolerance. Always consult with a healthcare provider before starting any new dietary supplement, especially if you have existing health conditions or concerns.

Pain Relief and Anti-Inflammatory Recipes

Castor Oil and Cayenne Pepper Pain Relief Cream

Beneficial effects

The Castor Oil and Cayenne Pepper Pain Relief Cream combines the potent anti-inflammatory and analgesic properties of castor oil with the warming sensation of cayenne pepper. This cream is designed to alleviate muscle aches, joint pain, and reduce inflammation, providing a natural and effective solution for pain relief.

Ingredients

- 2 tablespoons of cold-pressed castor oil
- 1 teaspoon of cayenne pepper powder
- 1/4 cup of coconut oil
- 2 tablespoons of beeswax pellets
- 5 drops of peppermint essential oil (optional for a cooling effect and to enhance pain relief)

Instructions

1. In a double boiler, melt the coconut oil and beeswax pellets together over low heat until fully dissolved and combined.
2. Carefully stir in the cayenne pepper powder and cold-pressed castor oil. Mix thoroughly to ensure the cayenne pepper is evenly distributed throughout the mixture.
3. Remove the mixture from heat and allow it to cool slightly. If using, add the peppermint essential oil at this stage and stir well.
4. Pour the mixture into a clean, dry container and allow it to solidify at room temperature.
5. Once solidified, close the container. Your pain relief cream is now ready for use.

Variations

- For an extra anti-inflammatory boost, add 5 drops of ginger essential oil to the mixture. Ginger enhances the pain-relieving properties of the cream.
- If you have sensitive skin, start with 1/2 teaspoon of cayenne pepper powder and adjust according to your tolerance level.

Storage tips

Store the cream in a cool, dry place away from direct sunlight. Ensure the container is tightly sealed to maintain the potency of the ingredients. The cream should remain effective for up to 6 months when stored properly.

Tips for allergens

If you are sensitive to cayenne pepper or peppermint oil, you can reduce the amount used or omit these ingredients. Always perform a patch test on a small area of your skin before applying the cream extensively, especially if you are trying new ingredients for the first time.

Castor Oil and Arnica Pain Relief Balm

Beneficial effects

The Castor Oil and Arnica Pain Relief Balm is a natural remedy designed to alleviate pain, reduce inflammation, and promote healing. Castor oil's anti-inflammatory properties work in synergy with arnica's analgesic effects to provide relief from muscle soreness, joint pain, and bruises. This balm is ideal for athletes, individuals with arthritis, or anyone seeking a natural alternative to synthetic pain relief creams.

Ingredients

- 1/4 cup cold-pressed castor oil
- 1/4 cup coconut oil
- 2 tablespoons beeswax pellets
- 2 tablespoons arnica montana flowers
- 10 drops of peppermint essential oil (optional for cooling effect and pain relief)

Instructions

1. Begin by melting the beeswax pellets and coconut oil together in a double boiler over low heat, stirring occasionally until fully melted.
2. Add the arnica montana flowers to the melted mixture and continue to simmer over low heat for 20-30 minutes, allowing the arnica to infuse into the oils.
3. Carefully strain the mixture to remove the arnica flowers, ensuring to press out as much oil as possible from the flowers.
4. Return the strained oil mixture to the double boiler and add the cold-pressed castor oil, stirring until well combined.
5. Remove from heat and let the mixture cool slightly before adding the peppermint essential oil, if using. Stir thoroughly to ensure even distribution of the essential oil.
6. Pour the balm into clean, dry containers and allow it to cool and solidify at room temperature.
7. Once solidified, close the containers. Your pain relief balm is ready for use.

Variations

- For extra anti-inflammatory benefits, add 5 drops of lavender essential oil to the mixture.
- If you prefer a vegan version, substitute beeswax with the same amount of candelilla wax.

Storage tips

Store the balm in a cool, dry place away from direct sunlight. If stored properly, the balm should remain effective for up to 12 months. Ensure the containers are tightly sealed to maintain the potency of the essential oils.

Tips for allergens

If you are sensitive to peppermint or any other essential oils, you can omit them from the recipe. Always perform a patch test on a small area of your skin before applying the balm extensively, especially if you have sensitive skin or are prone to allergies.

Castor Oil and St. John's Wort Anti-Inflammatory Oil

Beneficial effects

The Castor Oil and St. John's Wort Anti-Inflammatory Oil is crafted to provide relief from inflammation and pain associated with conditions like arthritis, muscle aches, and nerve pain. Castor oil, renowned for its anti-inflammatory properties, works in synergy with St. John's Wort, which has been traditionally used to soothe nerve pain and promote healing. This powerful combination helps to reduce swelling, ease discomfort, and support the body's natural healing processes.

Ingredients

- 2 tablespoons of cold-pressed castor oil
- 1 tablespoon of St. John's Wort oil
- 5 drops of lavender essential oil (optional for additional pain relief and a calming scent)

Instructions

1. In a clean glass bowl, mix the cold-pressed castor oil with the St. John's Wort oil until well combined.
2. If using, add the lavender essential oil to the oil blend and stir thoroughly. The lavender oil can enhance the anti-inflammatory effects and provide a soothing aroma.
3. Transfer the mixture to a dark glass bottle to protect the oils from light, which can degrade their therapeutic properties.
4. To use, apply a small amount of the oil to the affected area and gently massage in circular motions until fully absorbed. For best results, apply the oil 2-3 times daily, especially after a warm bath or shower to enhance absorption.

Variations

- For enhanced circulation and additional warmth, add 2 drops of ginger essential oil to the mixture. Ginger's warming properties can help increase blood flow to the area and provide additional pain relief.
- If you have sensitive skin, you can dilute the mixture further with an additional tablespoon of a carrier oil like almond or olive oil to minimize the risk of irritation.

Storage tips

Store the oil in a cool, dark place to maintain its potency. The dark glass bottle will help preserve the therapeutic qualities of the oils for up to 6 months. Ensure the bottle is tightly sealed after each use to prevent oxidation.

Tips for allergens

If you are sensitive to lavender or any other essential oils, you can omit them from the recipe. Always perform a patch test on a small area of your skin before using the oil extensively, especially if you have sensitive skin or are prone to allergies.

Castor Oil and Ginger Root Pain Relief Gel

Beneficial effects

The Castor Oil and Ginger Root Pain Relief Gel combines the potent anti-inflammatory properties of castor oil with the natural pain-relieving effects of ginger root. This gel is designed to alleviate muscle soreness, reduce inflammation, and provide targeted relief from joint pain. Castor oil penetrates deep into the skin to soothe discomfort, while ginger root increases circulation and warmth to the affected area, speeding up the healing process.

Ingredients

- 3 tablespoons of cold-pressed castor oil
- 2 tablespoons of freshly grated ginger root
- 1/4 cup of aloe vera gel
- 10 drops of peppermint essential oil

Instructions

1. In a small saucepan, gently heat the castor oil over low heat. Do not allow it to boil.
2. Add the freshly grated ginger root to the warm castor oil and simmer for 5 minutes to infuse the oil with ginger.
3. Strain the ginger pieces from the oil using a fine mesh sieve or cheesecloth, and discard the ginger.
4. Allow the infused castor oil to cool to room temperature.
5. In a mixing bowl, combine the cooled castor oil with the aloe vera gel. Mix thoroughly until well blended.
6. Add the peppermint essential oil to the mixture and stir to incorporate.
7. Transfer the gel to a clean, airtight container for storage.

Variations

- For an extra cooling effect, increase the amount of peppermint essential oil to 15 drops.
- If you prefer a thicker gel, add 1 teaspoon of xanthan gum to the mixture and blend until it reaches the desired consistency.

Storage tips

Store the pain relief gel in a cool, dark place. If stored properly in an airtight container, the gel can last for up to 2 weeks. For longer shelf life and additional cooling sensation upon application, store the gel in the refrigerator.

Tips for allergens

If you are allergic to peppermint, you can substitute it with lavender essential oil for its pain-relieving and anti-inflammatory properties. Always perform a patch test on a small area of your skin before using the gel extensively, especially if you have sensitive skin or are prone to allergies.

Castor Oil and Turmeric Anti-Inflammatory Paste

Beneficial effects

The Castor Oil and Turmeric Anti-Inflammatory Paste is a potent remedy designed to reduce inflammation, alleviate pain, and promote healing. This natural treatment harnesses the powerful anti-inflammatory properties of turmeric, combined with the soothing and moisturizing effects of castor oil, making it an effective solution for joint pain, skin irritations, and other inflammatory conditions.

Ingredients

- 2 tablespoons of cold-pressed castor oil
- 1 tablespoon of turmeric powder
- A few drops of water (to form a paste)

Instructions

1. In a small bowl, mix the turmeric powder with cold-pressed castor oil.
2. Add a few drops of water to the mixture, just enough to form a thick paste. Stir well to ensure all ingredients are fully combined.
3. Apply the paste directly to the affected area, gently massaging it into the skin.
4. Cover the area with a clean cloth or bandage and let it sit for 30 minutes to an hour.
5. Rinse off the paste with warm water and pat the skin dry with a soft towel.
6. Repeat this treatment 1-2 times daily as needed for pain relief and reduced inflammation.

Variations

- For enhanced pain relief, add a half teaspoon of ground ginger to the paste. Ginger's additional anti-inflammatory properties can further soothe discomfort.
- If you have sensitive skin, you can add more castor oil to dilute the turmeric and reduce the risk of irritation.

Storage tips

It's best to prepare the paste fresh for each use to ensure the potency of the turmeric. However, if you must prepare in advance, store the mixture in an airtight container in the refrigerator for up to 24 hours.

Tips for allergens

If you are allergic to turmeric or castor oil, conduct a patch test by applying a small amount of the paste to a discreet area of skin. If irritation occurs, discontinue use immediately. For those sensitive to ginger, omit this ingredient from the variations to avoid potential reactions.

Castor Oil and Black Pepper Pain Relief Lotion

Beneficial effects

The Castor Oil and Black Pepper Pain Relief Lotion is crafted to provide targeted relief from muscle pain, stiffness, and inflammation. Castor oil, renowned for its anti-inflammatory and analgesic properties, penetrates deep into the skin to soothe sore muscles and joints. Black pepper essential oil enhances circulation, offering warmth and further easing discomfort. This combination is ideal for those seeking natural pain relief options, reducing the need for synthetic medications and promoting a holistic approach to health.

Ingredients
- 1/4 cup cold-pressed castor oil
- 1/4 cup coconut oil
- 2 tablespoons beeswax pellets
- 10 drops black pepper essential oil
- 5 drops lavender essential oil (optional, for additional soothing effects)

Instructions
1. In a double boiler, melt the beeswax pellets and coconut oil together, stirring continuously until fully dissolved.
2. Remove the mixture from heat and allow it to cool slightly before adding the cold-pressed castor oil. Stir well to ensure all ingredients are evenly combined.
3. Add the black pepper essential oil to the mixture, and if using, the lavender essential oil. Mix thoroughly to distribute the oils throughout the lotion.
4. Pour the lotion into a clean, dry container and allow it to solidify at room temperature.
5. To use, massage a small amount of the lotion onto the affected areas. Apply 2-3 times daily or as needed for pain relief.

Variations
- For those with sensitive skin, reduce the amount of black pepper essential oil to 5 drops and increase lavender essential oil to 10 drops to mitigate sensitivity while still providing pain relief.
- To enhance the warming effect, add 5 drops of ginger essential oil to the mixture, known for its ability to soothe sore muscles and improve circulation.

Storage tips
Store the pain relief lotion in a cool, dark place to maintain its potency. Ensure the container is tightly sealed to prevent the lotion from drying out. When stored properly, the lotion can be used for up to 6 months.

Tips for allergens
If you are allergic to coconut oil, it can be substituted with jojoba oil, which is hypoallergenic and also beneficial for skin health. Always perform a patch test on a small area of your skin before applying the lotion extensively, especially if incorporating new essential oils into your routine.

Castor Oil and Frankincense Pain Relief Serum

Beneficial effects
The Castor Oil and Frankincense Pain Relief Serum is an all-natural solution designed to alleviate chronic pain, reduce inflammation, and promote healing. Castor oil, renowned for its anti-inflammatory properties,

works in synergy with frankincense, known for its ability to relieve joint pain, reduce arthritis symptoms, and support the immune system. This serum offers a holistic approach to pain management without the side effects associated with synthetic painkillers.

Ingredients
- 3 tablespoons of cold-pressed castor oil
- 10 drops of frankincense essential oil
- 2 tablespoons of almond oil (as a carrier oil)
- Small glass bottle with dropper

Instructions
1. In a clean bowl, mix the cold-pressed castor oil with the almond oil thoroughly. The almond oil serves as a carrier, facilitating the application and absorption of the serum.
2. Add the frankincense essential oil to the oil mixture and stir well to ensure all ingredients are evenly blended.
3. Using a funnel, carefully transfer the serum into the glass dropper bottle.
4. To apply, place a few drops of the serum on your fingertips and gently massage into the affected area. Focus on areas with muscle soreness, joint pain, or inflammation.
5. Use the serum twice daily, in the morning and evening, for best results.

Variations
- For additional analgesic properties, add 5 drops of lavender essential oil to the mixture. Lavender will not only enhance the serum's pain-relieving capabilities but also provide a calming scent.
- If you have sensitive skin, you can substitute almond oil with jojoba oil, which is lighter and less likely to cause irritation.

Storage tips
Store the pain relief serum in a cool, dark place to preserve the potency of the essential oils. Ensure the dropper bottle is tightly sealed to prevent oxidation. When stored properly, the serum should remain effective for up to 6 months.

Tips for allergens
If you are allergic to almond oil, substituting it with coconut oil or olive oil can provide similar benefits without the risk of an allergic reaction. Always perform a patch test on a small area of your skin before using the serum extensively, especially if you're incorporating new ingredients into your regimen.

Castor Oil and Helichrysum Pain Relief Oil

Beneficial effects
The Castor Oil and Helichrysum Pain Relief Oil is a natural remedy designed to alleviate pain, reduce inflammation, and accelerate healing. Castor oil's anti-inflammatory properties work in synergy with helichrysum essential oil, known for its ability to promote tissue regeneration and soothe discomfort. This

powerful combination is particularly effective for joint pain, muscle aches, bruises, and sprains, offering a holistic approach to pain management without the side effects associated with synthetic medications.

Ingredients
- 2 tablespoons of cold-pressed castor oil
- 10 drops of helichrysum essential oil
- 1 tablespoon of jojoba oil (as a carrier oil)

Instructions
1. In a clean glass bottle, combine the cold-pressed castor oil with jojoba oil. Jojoba oil is used as a carrier to dilute the essential oil and facilitate application.
2. Add the helichrysum essential oil to the oil mixture. Cap the bottle and shake well to ensure the oils are thoroughly blended.
3. To use, apply a small amount of the pain relief oil to the affected area.
4. Gently massage the oil into the skin with circular motions until it is fully absorbed.
5. For best results, apply the oil 2-3 times daily to the affected area until symptoms improve.

Variations
- For enhanced pain relief, add 5 drops of lavender essential oil to the mixture. Lavender adds additional anti-inflammatory and soothing properties.
- If treating a larger area or for a more spreadable consistency, increase the amount of jojoba oil to 2 tablespoons.

Storage tips
Store the pain relief oil in a cool, dark place to preserve the potency of the essential oils. Ensure the bottle is tightly sealed to prevent oxidation. When stored properly, the oil can remain effective for up to 6 months.

Tips for allergens
If you are sensitive to helichrysum or jojoba oil, perform a patch test on a small area of your skin before widespread use. Should you experience any adverse reaction, discontinue use immediately. For those allergic to jojoba oil, it can be substituted with sweet almond oil or coconut oil as alternative carrier oils.

Castor Oil and Marjoram Pain Relief Rub

Beneficial effects
The Castor Oil and Marjoram Pain Relief Rub is designed to alleviate joint pain, muscle soreness, and inflammation. Castor oil's anti-inflammatory properties work to reduce swelling and discomfort, while marjoram essential oil is known for its ability to soothe muscle spasms and tension. Together, they create a powerful remedy that not only eases pain but also promotes relaxation and well-being.

Ingredients
- 3 tablespoons of cold-pressed castor oil
- 10 drops of marjoram essential oil

- 2 tablespoons of beeswax (optional, for a thicker consistency)
- 1 tablespoon of coconut oil (to enhance absorption)

Instructions

1. If you're using beeswax for a thicker rub, start by melting it over low heat in a double boiler.
2. Once melted, stir in the coconut oil until well combined.
3. Remove from heat and allow the mixture to cool slightly before adding the castor oil. Mix thoroughly.
4. Add the marjoram essential oil to the mixture, stirring well to ensure it's evenly distributed.
5. Pour the mixture into a clean, dry container and allow it to solidify. If you skipped the beeswax, simply mix the castor oil, coconut oil, and marjoram essential oil in a bowl and transfer to a container.
6. To use, massage a small amount of the pain relief rub into the affected areas. Apply with gentle, circular motions to enhance absorption and blood flow.

Variations

- For additional analgesic properties, add 5 drops of peppermint essential oil to the mixture. Peppermint oil can provide a cooling sensation that further relieves pain.
- If you prefer a vegan option, substitute beeswax with an equal amount of candelilla wax.

Storage tips

Store the pain relief rub in a cool, dark place to preserve its potency. If you've added beeswax, the balm will have a longer shelf life compared to the oil mixture alone. Ensure the container is tightly sealed to prevent leakage and contamination.

Tips for allergens

If you have sensitive skin or are allergic to any of the ingredients, perform a patch test on a small area of skin before applying the rub extensively. Substitute marjoram essential oil with lavender essential oil for a gentler alternative if needed.

Castor Oil and Boswellia Pain Relief Cream

Beneficial effects

The Castor Oil and Boswellia Pain Relief Cream is a natural remedy formulated to alleviate pain and reduce inflammation. This cream combines the anti-inflammatory properties of castor oil with the analgesic benefits of Boswellia, making it effective for joint pain, arthritis, and muscle aches. Castor oil penetrates deep into the skin, delivering the therapeutic compounds directly to the affected areas, while Boswellia, also known as Indian Frankincense, has been shown to decrease inflammation and provide pain relief.

Ingredients

- 2 tablespoons of cold-pressed castor oil
- 2 tablespoons of Boswellia serrata extract
- 1/4 cup of coconut oil

- 2 tablespoons of beeswax pellets
- 10 drops of lavender essential oil (optional for additional anti-inflammatory and soothing effects)

Instructions

1. In a double boiler, gently melt the coconut oil and beeswax pellets together until fully combined.
2. Remove the mixture from heat and allow it to cool slightly.
3. Stir in the cold-pressed castor oil and Boswellia serrata extract until the mixture is well blended.
4. If using, add the lavender essential oil to the mixture for its calming and anti-inflammatory properties.
5. Pour the mixture into a clean, dry container and allow it to cool and solidify.
6. Once solidified, the pain relief cream is ready to use. Apply a small amount to the affected area and massage gently until fully absorbed. Use 2-3 times daily or as needed for pain relief.

Variations

- For enhanced pain relief, add 5 drops of peppermint essential oil to the mixture. Peppermint oil contains menthol, which provides a cooling sensation and further helps to relieve pain.
- If you prefer a vegan option, substitute beeswax with an equal amount of candelilla wax.

Storage tips

Store the pain relief cream in a cool, dry place, away from direct sunlight. If stored properly in an airtight container, the cream should remain effective for up to 6 months.

Tips for allergens

If you are sensitive to lavender or peppermint essential oil, you can omit these from the recipe without significantly affecting the pain-relieving properties of the cream. Always perform a patch test on a small area of your skin before applying the cream extensively, especially if you have sensitive skin or are prone to allergies.

Immune System Remedies

Castor Oil and Echinacea Immune Booster

Beneficial effects
The Castor Oil and Echinacea Immune Booster is designed to enhance the body's natural defense mechanisms, promoting a healthy immune system. Castor oil, with its anti-inflammatory and antibacterial properties, works to support the body's lymphatic drainage, thereby improving immune function. Echinacea, a herb renowned for its immune-boosting capabilities, aids in fighting off infections and reducing the duration of colds and flu. This potent combination offers a natural way to bolster the immune system, especially during times of increased stress or susceptibility to illness.

Ingredients
- 2 tablespoons of cold-pressed castor oil
- 1 cup of echinacea tea (cooled)
- 1 teaspoon of honey (optional, for taste)
- 1/4 teaspoon of lemon juice (optional, for vitamin C boost)

Instructions
1. Prepare the echinacea tea according to package instructions and allow it to cool to room temperature.
2. Mix the cold-pressed castor oil into the cooled echinacea tea, stirring until well combined.
3. If desired, add honey to sweeten and lemon juice for an additional vitamin C boost. Stir thoroughly to ensure all ingredients are evenly mixed.
4. Consume the mixture once daily, preferably in the morning, to support immune health.

Variations
- For an added antioxidant boost, include a pinch of ground turmeric or ginger to the mixture. Both spices are known for their immune-supporting properties.
- If echinacea tea is not available, you can substitute it with green tea, which also has immune-boosting effects.

Storage tips
It's best to prepare this immune booster fresh each time for optimal benefits. However, if you need to make it ahead of time, store the mixture in the refrigerator for up to 24 hours. Ensure to stir well before consuming.

Tips for allergens
If you are allergic to echinacea, you can replace it with elderberry syrup, another potent immune-supporting substitute. Always ensure that you are not allergic to any of the ingredients by performing a patch test or consulting with a healthcare provider before incorporating this immune booster into your routine.

Castor Oil and Elderberry Immune Syrup

Beneficial effects

The Castor Oil and Elderberry Immune Syrup is a potent blend aimed at boosting the immune system, fighting off colds and flu, and providing antioxidant support. Castor oil serves as a powerful anti-inflammatory agent, while elderberries are renowned for their immune-boosting properties and high levels of vitamins and antioxidants. This syrup is ideal for those looking to enhance their immune response naturally and protect themselves during cold and flu season.

Ingredients

- 2 tablespoons of cold-pressed castor oil
- 1/2 cup of dried elderberries
- 3 cups of water
- 1 cup of raw honey
- 1 cinnamon stick
- 5 cloves
- 1 piece of fresh ginger, sliced

Instructions

1. Combine the dried elderberries, water, cinnamon stick, cloves, and ginger in a medium saucepan.
2. Bring the mixture to a boil, then reduce the heat and simmer for about 45 minutes to an hour, or until the liquid has reduced by half.
3. Remove from heat and let the mixture cool until it is warm to the touch.
4. Strain the liquid through a fine mesh sieve or cheesecloth, pressing on the berries to extract as much liquid as possible. Discard the solids.
5. Once the liquid has cooled to lukewarm, stir in the cold-pressed castor oil and raw honey until well combined.
6. Transfer the syrup to a clean, sterilized glass bottle or jar.

Variations

- For an extra immune boost, add 1/2 teaspoon of ground turmeric to the simmering mixture.
- If you prefer a vegan version, substitute the honey with maple syrup or agave nectar, though keep in mind this will alter the flavor slightly.

Storage tips

Store the immune syrup in the refrigerator. It will keep for up to two months when stored properly. Make sure the bottle or jar is tightly sealed to maintain freshness and potency.

Tips for allergens

If you are allergic to any of the spices used in this recipe, they can be omitted without significantly affecting the immune-boosting properties of the syrup. Always ensure that you source high-quality, pure castor oil that is safe for internal use, and consult with a healthcare provider if you have any concerns or existing health conditions.

Castor Oil and Astragalus Root Tonic

Beneficial effects
The Castor Oil and Astragalus Root Tonic is a powerful blend aimed at enhancing the immune system, providing anti-inflammatory benefits, and supporting overall wellness. Castor oil, with its immune-boosting properties, works in harmony with astragalus root, a well-known adaptogen that increases the body's resistance to stress and disease. This tonic is particularly beneficial during seasonal changes or times of high stress when the immune system needs extra support.

Ingredients
- 2 tablespoons of cold-pressed castor oil
- 1 tablespoon of dried astragalus root
- 1 cup of boiling water
- Honey or lemon to taste (optional)

Instructions
1. Place the dried astragalus root in a heat-proof container or teapot.
2. Pour 1 cup of boiling water over the astragalus root and cover. Allow it to steep for 15-20 minutes to extract the beneficial compounds.
3. Strain the astragalus root from the water and let the tea cool to a comfortable drinking temperature.
4. Stir in 2 tablespoons of cold-pressed castor oil into the astragalus tea until well combined.
5. If desired, add honey or lemon to taste for flavor enhancement.
6. Consume the tonic once daily, preferably in the morning, to boost the immune system and promote overall health.

Variations
- For added immune support, include a teaspoon of echinacea tincture to the tonic. Echinacea is another powerful herb known for its immune-enhancing properties.
- If the taste of castor oil is too strong, mix the tonic with a small amount of natural fruit juice to improve palatability.

Storage tips
It's best to prepare this tonic fresh each time for maximum efficacy. However, the astragalus tea (without castor oil) can be made in advance and stored in the refrigerator for up to 48 hours. Add castor oil to individual servings as needed.

Tips for allergens
If you have a sensitivity or allergy to astragalus, consult with a healthcare provider before adding this tonic to your routine. For those allergic to honey, it can be omitted or substituted with maple syrup as a sweetener.

Castor Oil and Garlic Immune Elixir

Beneficial effects

The Castor Oil and Garlic Immune Elixir is crafted to bolster the immune system, leveraging the potent antimicrobial properties of garlic and the anti-inflammatory benefits of castor oil. This elixir is designed to support the body's natural defenses against pathogens, promote healthy lymphatic drainage, and enhance overall well-being. Regular consumption can help ward off common colds, reduce inflammation, and maintain a balanced immune response.

Ingredients

- 2 tablespoons of cold-pressed castor oil
- 1 clove of fresh garlic, minced
- 1 cup of warm water
- 1 teaspoon of honey (optional, for taste)
- A squeeze of lemon juice (optional, for vitamin C boost)

Instructions

1. Place the minced garlic in a cup of warm water and let it steep for 5-10 minutes.
2. Strain the garlic from the water, ensuring to press out all the garlic juice.
3. Stir in the cold-pressed castor oil into the garlic-infused water.
4. If desired, add honey for sweetness and lemon juice for an added vitamin C boost. Mix well until all components are thoroughly combined.
5. Consume the elixir on an empty stomach in the morning to maximize its immune-boosting effects.

Variations

- For those sensitive to the taste of garlic, adding a pinch of ground ginger can help mask the flavor while adding additional anti-inflammatory and immune-boosting properties.
- If you prefer not to consume castor oil directly, you can substitute it with olive oil, which also has immune-supporting benefits.

Storage tips

It's best to prepare this elixir fresh each morning to ensure the potency of the garlic and castor oil. However, if you need to prepare it in advance, store it in the refrigerator for no more than 24 hours to maintain freshness. Use a sealed glass container to prevent odors from permeating.

Tips for allergens

If you are allergic to honey, you can omit it from the recipe or substitute it with maple syrup. For those with a sensitivity to citrus, the lemon juice can be left out without significantly affecting the immune-boosting properties of the elixir. Always perform a patch test on your skin with diluted castor oil and garlic juice to ensure there is no adverse reaction before consuming the elixir.

Castor Oil and Ginger Immune Tea

Beneficial effects

The Castor Oil and Ginger Immune Tea is a warming and soothing beverage designed to boost the immune system and alleviate symptoms of cold and flu. Castor oil, with its anti-inflammatory properties, aids in reducing inflammation and supporting the body's natural defense mechanisms. Ginger, known for its potent antiviral and antibacterial properties, helps in fighting infections and soothing sore throats, making this tea an excellent remedy for enhancing immune health and providing comfort during illness.

Ingredients

- 1 tablespoon of cold-pressed castor oil
- 1 inch of fresh ginger root, grated
- 1 tablespoon of honey (optional, for sweetness and additional antibacterial properties)
- 1 cup of boiling water
- Juice of half a lemon (optional, for vitamin C and flavor)

Instructions

1. Place the grated ginger in a mug or teapot.
2. Pour the boiling water over the ginger and allow it to steep for 5-10 minutes.
3. Strain the ginger pieces from the tea and pour the tea into a mug if using a teapot.
4. Stir in the cold-pressed castor oil until it is well integrated into the tea.
5. If desired, add honey and lemon juice to taste, and stir well to combine.
6. Drink the tea while it is still warm to maximize its soothing and immune-boosting effects.

Variations

- For an extra immune boost, add a pinch of ground turmeric to the tea while it steeps. Turmeric's curcumin content offers powerful anti-inflammatory and antioxidant benefits.
- If you prefer a spicier tea, include a pinch of cayenne pepper, which can help clear nasal congestion and increase circulation.

Storage tips

This tea is best enjoyed fresh to ensure the potency of its ingredients. However, the ginger can be steeped in advance and stored in the refrigerator for up to 24 hours. Warm the tea and add the castor oil, honey, and lemon juice just before drinking.

Tips for allergens

If you are allergic to honey, you can omit it or substitute it with maple syrup. Always ensure that you are not allergic to any of the ingredients by performing a patch test or consulting with a healthcare provider before incorporating this tea into your routine.

Castor Oil and Turmeric Immune Paste

Beneficial effects

The Castor Oil and Turmeric Immune Paste is a potent blend designed to boost the immune system, reduce inflammation, and fight off pathogens. Castor oil's ricinoleic acid has anti-inflammatory and antimicrobial properties, while turmeric, with its active compound curcumin, is known for its powerful antioxidant and immune-boosting effects. This combination makes the paste an excellent preventive measure against common illnesses and a supportive treatment for maintaining overall health.

Ingredients

- 2 tablespoons of cold-pressed castor oil
- 1 tablespoon of turmeric powder
- 1/2 teaspoon of black pepper (to enhance curcumin absorption)
- 1 tablespoon of honey (for taste and additional antimicrobial properties)
- 1/4 cup of warm water

Instructions

1. In a small bowl, combine the turmeric powder and black pepper.
2. Add the cold-pressed castor oil to the turmeric and pepper mixture, stirring until a smooth paste forms.
3. Gradually mix in the honey, ensuring it's well incorporated into the paste.
4. Slowly add the warm water to the mixture, stirring continuously to achieve a consistent paste.
5. Consume 1 teaspoon of the immune paste daily, preferably in the morning on an empty stomach, to boost immunity and promote overall health.

Variations

- For those with a sensitive palate, adjust the amount of honey to sweeten the paste to your liking.
- To make the paste more potent, add a teaspoon of ginger powder for its additional anti-inflammatory and immune-boosting properties.

Storage tips

Store any unused portion of the immune paste in an airtight container in the refrigerator. Use within 5 days for optimal freshness and efficacy.

Tips for allergens

If you are allergic to honey, you can substitute it with maple syrup or simply omit it. For individuals sensitive to black pepper, start with a smaller amount and adjust according to tolerance. Always ensure you're not allergic to any of the ingredients by performing a patch test before consuming the paste regularly.

Castor Oil and Lemon Immune Drink

Beneficial effects

The Castor Oil and Lemon Immune Drink is crafted to enhance the immune system, detoxify the body, and provide a boost of energy. Castor oil, with its anti-inflammatory and antimicrobial properties, aids in improving lymphatic circulation and supporting immune function. Lemon, rich in Vitamin C and antioxidants, helps in fighting off infections and detoxifying the liver. This drink is ideal for those looking to naturally bolster their immune system and improve overall health.

Ingredients

- 1 tablespoon of cold-pressed, hexane-free castor oil
- Juice of 1/2 organic lemon
- 1 cup of warm water
- 1 teaspoon of organic honey (optional, for taste)

Instructions

1. Warm the water to a comfortable drinking temperature and pour it into a glass.
2. Squeeze the juice of half a lemon into the warm water.
3. Add the tablespoon of cold-pressed, hexane-free castor oil to the lemon water.
4. If desired, add a teaspoon of organic honey to sweeten and mix well until all ingredients are fully combined.
5. Drink this immune-boosting mixture first thing in the morning on an empty stomach to maximize its benefits.

Variations

- For an extra immune boost, add a pinch of ground turmeric or ginger to the drink. Both spices have powerful anti-inflammatory and antioxidant properties.
- If you prefer a cooler beverage, allow the mixture to cool to room temperature before drinking, or add a few ice cubes.

Storage tips

Prepare the Castor Oil and Lemon Immune Drink fresh each morning to ensure the potency of the ingredients. It is not recommended to store the mixture as the lemon juice and castor oil are most effective when consumed immediately after preparation.

Tips for allergens

If you are sensitive to honey, you can easily omit it from the recipe without affecting the immune-boosting properties of the drink. Always ensure that the castor oil used is cold-pressed and hexane-free to avoid potential irritants and maximize health benefits.

Castor Oil and Honey Immune Support

Beneficial effects

The Castor Oil and Honey Immune Support concoction is designed to bolster the body's natural defenses, providing a nurturing blend of antibacterial, anti-inflammatory, and antioxidant properties. Castor oil, known for its immune-boosting capabilities, works in tandem with honey's natural antioxidants and antibacterial agents to strengthen the immune system, making this remedy especially beneficial during cold and flu season or whenever extra immune support is needed.

Ingredients

- 2 tablespoons of cold-pressed castor oil
- 2 tablespoons of raw, organic honey
- 1 cup of warm water
- Juice of 1/2 lemon (optional, for added vitamin C and flavor)

Instructions

1. Warm the water to a comfortable drinking temperature.
2. Combine the warm water with the cold-pressed castor oil in a glass, stirring thoroughly to mix.
3. Add the raw, organic honey to the mixture and stir until it is completely dissolved.
4. If using, squeeze in the juice of half a lemon and stir again to incorporate.
5. Consume this mixture once daily, preferably in the morning on an empty stomach, to support immune health.

Variations

- For an added boost, include a pinch of ground cinnamon or turmeric to the mixture. Both spices have anti-inflammatory properties and can enhance the immune-supporting effects.
- If you prefer a cold beverage, mix all the ingredients in cold water and add a few ice cubes for a refreshing immune-supporting drink.

Storage tips

It's best to prepare this immune support drink fresh each time to ensure the potency of the ingredients. However, if you need to prepare it in advance, store the mixture in the refrigerator for no more than 24 hours to maintain freshness.

Tips for allergens

If you are allergic to honey, you can substitute it with maple syrup, which also contains antioxidants but ensure it's pure and organic. Always check for any known allergies to the ingredients used, and consult with a healthcare provider if unsure.

Castor Oil and Ginseng Immune Tonic

Beneficial effects

The Castor Oil and Ginseng Immune Tonic is formulated to enhance immune function, increase energy levels, and improve overall wellness. Castor oil, with its anti-inflammatory and antimicrobial properties, supports the body's natural defense mechanisms, while ginseng is renowned for its immune-boosting and vitality-enhancing effects. This tonic is especially beneficial during times of stress, fatigue, or when extra immune support is needed.

Ingredients

- 2 tablespoons of cold-pressed castor oil
- 1 teaspoon of ginseng extract
- 1 cup of warm water
- Honey or lemon to taste (optional, for flavor)

Instructions

1. Warm the water to a comfortable drinking temperature.
2. Mix the cold-pressed castor oil and ginseng extract into the warm water, stirring until well combined.
3. Add honey or lemon to taste, if desired, and stir again to incorporate.
4. Consume the tonic first thing in the morning on an empty stomach to maximize absorption and benefits.

Variations

- For an added boost, include a pinch of ground turmeric or ginger to the tonic. Both spices have anti-inflammatory properties and can enhance the immune-supporting effects of the tonic.
- If the taste of castor oil is too strong, reduce the amount to 1 tablespoon and gradually increase as you become accustomed to the flavor.

Storage tips

Prepare this tonic fresh each time to ensure the effectiveness of the ingredients. It is not recommended to store any prepared mixture as the active properties are best when fresh.

Tips for allergens

If you have a sensitivity or allergy to ginseng, start with a smaller dose to ensure no adverse reactions occur. Always consult with a healthcare provider before adding new supplements to your routine, especially if you have existing health conditions or are taking medication.

Castor Oil and Oregano Oil Immune Drops

Beneficial effects

The Castor Oil and Oregano Oil Immune Drops are a potent combination designed to boost the immune system and provide antimicrobial benefits. Castor oil, with its anti-inflammatory properties, supports the body's natural defense mechanisms, while oregano oil, known for its powerful antibacterial and antiviral qualities, helps to fight off pathogens and infections. Together, they form a natural remedy that can enhance immune function, protect against illness, and promote overall wellness.

Ingredients

- 2 tablespoons of cold-pressed castor oil
- 5 drops of oregano essential oil
- 1 tablespoon of honey (optional, for taste and additional antimicrobial properties)
- 1 cup of warm water

Instructions

1. Add the cold-pressed castor oil to a glass of warm water.
2. Incorporate the oregano essential oil into the mixture, ensuring it's well dispersed.
3. If desired, add a tablespoon of honey to the mixture for sweetness and its natural antimicrobial properties. Stir the mixture thoroughly until all ingredients are combined.
4. Consume the immune drops first thing in the morning on an empty stomach to maximize absorption and benefits.
5. Repeat daily, especially during cold and flu season, to support the immune system.

Variations

- For those sensitive to the taste of oregano oil, reduce the amount to 2-3 drops and gradually increase as tolerated.
- To enhance the immune-boosting effects, add a squeeze of fresh lemon juice to the mixture for an additional dose of vitamin C.

Storage tips

Prepare the immune drops fresh each morning to ensure the potency of the oregano oil and the freshness of the other ingredients. It is not recommended to store any premade mixture as the essential oil may lose its effectiveness over time.

Tips for allergens

If you have a sensitivity or allergy to oregano oil, start with a lower dose to assess tolerance. For individuals allergic to honey, it can be omitted without significantly affecting the immune-boosting properties of the drops. Always consult with a healthcare provider before starting any new dietary supplement, especially if you have existing health conditions or are taking medications.

Detox Cleansing Recipes

Castor Oil and Lemon Detox Cleanse

Beneficial effects

The Castor Oil and Lemon Detox Cleanse is designed to support the body's natural detoxification processes, aiding in the removal of toxins and promoting liver health. Castor oil's anti-inflammatory properties help soothe the digestive system, while lemon juice, rich in vitamin C, boosts the immune system and aids in digestion. This cleanse can help improve energy levels, promote clearer skin, and support overall well-being.

Ingredients
- 2 tablespoons of cold-pressed castor oil
- Juice of 1 organic lemon
- 1 cup of warm water

Instructions
1. Warm the water to a comfortable drinking temperature.
2. Squeeze the juice of one lemon into the warm water.
3. Add the cold-pressed castor oil to the lemon water and stir well to combine.
4. Drink the mixture first thing in the morning on an empty stomach.
5. Wait at least 30 minutes before consuming breakfast.

Variations
- To enhance the detoxifying effects, add a pinch of cayenne pepper to the mixture. Cayenne pepper is known for its ability to boost circulation and aid in the elimination of toxins.
- For those who prefer a sweeter taste, add a teaspoon of raw honey to the mixture. Honey adds antibacterial properties and can make the cleanse more palatable.

Storage tips

Prepare the Castor Oil and Lemon Detox Cleanse fresh each morning to ensure the effectiveness of the ingredients. It is not recommended to store the mixture as the properties of lemon juice and castor oil are best when fresh.

Tips for allergens

If you have a sensitivity to citrus, start with a smaller amount of lemon juice and gradually increase it to assess tolerance. Always consult with a healthcare provider before starting any new detox regimen, especially if you have existing health conditions or concerns.

Castor Oil and Apple Cider Vinegar Detox Drink

Beneficial effects
The Castor Oil and Apple Cider Vinegar Detox Drink is a powerful detoxifying blend that aids in cleansing the liver, improving digestion, and supporting overall detoxification processes in the body. Castor oil, with its ability to support lymphatic drainage and liver function, combined with apple cider vinegar's properties of balancing pH levels and promoting gut health, makes this drink a potent tool for those looking to naturally detoxify their system and enhance their body's natural cleansing abilities.

Ingredients
- 2 tablespoons of cold-pressed castor oil
- 2 tablespoons of organic apple cider vinegar
- 1 cup of warm water
- 1 teaspoon of organic honey (optional, for sweetness)

Instructions
1. Warm the water to a comfortable drinking temperature.
2. In a glass, combine the warm water with the cold-pressed castor oil and organic apple cider vinegar.
3. Stir the mixture well to ensure the castor oil and apple cider vinegar are fully dispersed in the water.
4. If desired, add a teaspoon of organic honey to the mixture and stir until it dissolves completely. This step is optional but can improve the taste of the detox drink.
5. Consume the detox drink first thing in the morning on an empty stomach.

Variations
- For an added detox boost, include a squeeze of fresh lemon juice into the drink. Lemon juice can enhance the detoxifying effects and provide additional vitamin C.
- If you prefer a spicier kick, add a pinch of cayenne pepper to the mixture. Cayenne pepper is known for its metabolism-boosting properties and can complement the detox process.

Storage tips
It's best to prepare this detox drink fresh each morning to ensure the effectiveness of the ingredients. However, if you need to prepare it ahead of time, store it in the refrigerator for no more than 24 hours. Shake well before consuming.

Tips for allergens
If you are sensitive to honey, you can omit it from the recipe or substitute it with maple syrup for a vegan-friendly sweetener. Always ensure that you are not allergic to any of the ingredients by performing a patch test or consulting with a healthcare provider before incorporating this detox drink into your routine.

Castor Oil and Green Tea Detox Smoothie

Beneficial effects

The Castor Oil and Green Tea Detox Smoothie is designed to cleanse and rejuvenate the body by combining the detoxifying properties of green tea with the healing and anti-inflammatory benefits of castor oil. This smoothie aids in flushing out toxins, supporting liver function, and providing a rich source of antioxidants to combat oxidative stress, making it an ideal choice for those looking to boost their overall health and wellness.

Ingredients

- 1 tablespoon of cold-pressed castor oil
- 1 cup of brewed green tea, cooled
- 1/2 cup of fresh spinach leaves
- 1/2 a medium cucumber, sliced
- 1/2 an apple, cored and sliced
- Juice of 1/2 a lemon
- 1 tablespoon of honey (optional, for sweetness)

Instructions

1. Brew a cup of green tea and allow it to cool to room temperature.
2. In a blender, combine the cooled green tea, cold-pressed castor oil, spinach leaves, cucumber slices, apple slices, and lemon juice.
3. Blend on high until the mixture is smooth and well combined.
4. Taste the smoothie and, if desired, add honey for sweetness. Blend again briefly to mix in the honey.
5. Pour the smoothie into a glass and enjoy immediately for the best detoxifying effects.

Variations

- For an extra boost of fiber and antioxidants, add a tablespoon of ground flaxseed or chia seeds to the blender before mixing.
- If you prefer a creamier texture, include a 1/4 cup of Greek yogurt or a banana for added thickness and nutrients.

Storage tips

This detox smoothie is best enjoyed fresh to maximize the benefits of its ingredients. However, if you need to store it, keep the smoothie in an airtight container in the refrigerator for up to 24 hours. Shake well before drinking as separation may occur.

Tips for allergens

If you are allergic to any of the fruits or vegetables listed, they can be substituted with other non-allergenic options that provide similar health benefits. For those with a sensitivity to honey, it can be omitted or replaced with another natural sweetener like maple syrup.

Castor Oil and Ginger Detox Elixir

Beneficial effects

The Castor Oil and Ginger Detox Elixir is designed to cleanse the body, stimulate digestion, and support the immune system. Castor oil's anti-inflammatory properties help soothe the digestive tract, while ginger's antioxidant and anti-inflammatory effects aid in detoxification and promote gastrointestinal health. This elixir can help alleviate symptoms of bloating, indigestion, and nausea, making it an excellent choice for those looking to naturally detoxify their body and boost digestive health.

Ingredients

- 2 tablespoons of cold-pressed castor oil
- 1 tablespoon of freshly grated ginger
- 1 cup of hot water
- 1 teaspoon of lemon juice
- 1 teaspoon of honey (optional, for sweetness)

Instructions

1. Steep the freshly grated ginger in 1 cup of hot water for about 10 minutes.
2. Strain the ginger pieces from the water and let the ginger tea cool to a warm, drinkable temperature.
3. Stir in the cold-pressed castor oil and lemon juice into the ginger tea.
4. Add honey to taste, if desired, and mix well until all the ingredients are fully combined.
5. Consume the detox elixir in the morning on an empty stomach to maximize its detoxifying benefits.

Variations

- For an added detox boost, include a pinch of cayenne pepper to the elixir. Cayenne pepper has metabolism-boosting properties and can help increase the detoxification process.
- If you prefer a milder flavor, you can reduce the amount of ginger to 1/2 tablespoon and gradually increase it as your palate adjusts.

Storage tips

This elixir is best consumed fresh to ensure the potency of its ingredients. However, if you need to prepare it in advance, store it in the refrigerator for no more than 24 hours. Shake well before consuming.

Tips for allergens

If you are allergic to honey, you can substitute it with maple syrup or simply omit the sweetener altogether. For those sensitive to lemon or ginger, start with smaller amounts and adjust according to your tolerance. Always consult with a healthcare provider before starting any detox regimen, especially if you have existing health conditions or concerns.

Castor Oil and Turmeric Detox Tonic

Beneficial effects

The Castor Oil and Turmeric Detox Tonic is a powerful blend designed to cleanse the body, reduce inflammation, and support liver function. This tonic leverages the detoxifying properties of castor oil with the anti-inflammatory benefits of turmeric, making it an ideal remedy for promoting overall health and wellness. Regular consumption can help in flushing out toxins, easing digestive issues, and enhancing the body's natural detoxification processes.

Ingredients

- 2 tablespoons of cold-pressed castor oil
- 1/2 teaspoon of turmeric powder
- 1 cup of warm water
- Honey or lemon to taste (optional)

Instructions

1. Warm the water to a comfortable drinking temperature.
2. Add the turmeric powder to the warm water and stir until it is completely dissolved.
3. Stir in the cold-pressed castor oil, ensuring it is well mixed with the turmeric water.
4. If desired, add honey or lemon to taste, and mix well.
5. Consume this tonic first thing in the morning on an empty stomach to maximize its detoxifying effects.

Variations

- For an added immune boost, include a pinch of black pepper to the tonic. Piperine, found in black pepper, enhances the absorption of curcumin from turmeric.
- If the taste of castor oil is too strong, mix the tonic with a small amount of apple juice to improve palatability.

Storage tips

Prepare this tonic fresh each morning to ensure the effectiveness of the ingredients. It is not recommended to store the mixture as the active properties of turmeric and castor oil are best when fresh.

Tips for allergens

If you have a sensitivity or allergy to turmeric, start with a smaller dose to ensure no adverse reactions occur. Always consult with a healthcare provider before starting any new health regimen, especially if you have existing health conditions or are taking medication.

Castor Oil and Aloe Vera Detox Juice

Beneficial effects

The Castor Oil and Aloe Vera Detox Juice is a rejuvenating beverage designed to cleanse the body, hydrate the skin, and support digestive health. Castor oil's lymphatic-supportive properties aid in detoxification, while aloe vera's high content of vitamins, minerals, and amino acids nourishes and soothes the digestive tract, promoting overall wellness.

Ingredients

- 2 tablespoons of cold-pressed, hexane-free castor oil
- 1/2 cup of pure aloe vera juice
- 1 cup of fresh cucumber juice
- Juice of 1 lemon
- 1 tablespoon of honey (optional)
- 2 cups of water

Instructions

1. In a large pitcher, combine the aloe vera juice, cucumber juice, lemon juice, and water. Stir well to mix.
2. Add the cold-pressed, hexane-free castor oil to the juice mixture. Stir vigorously to ensure the oil is well incorporated.
3. If using, stir in the honey to sweeten the detox juice.
4. Refrigerate the mixture for at least 1 hour to chill.
5. Stir the detox juice well before serving. Consume 1 glass of the juice in the morning on an empty stomach for best detoxifying results.

Variations

- For an added detox boost, include a pinch of cayenne pepper or ginger powder to the juice mixture.
- If you prefer a smoothie-like consistency, blend the ingredients instead of stirring and add a handful of fresh spinach or kale.

Storage tips

The Castor Oil and Aloe Vera Detox Juice is best consumed fresh. However, it can be stored in the refrigerator for up to 24 hours. Ensure the pitcher is covered to maintain freshness and prevent absorption of other flavors from the fridge.

Tips for allergens

If you are allergic to any of the ingredients, they can be omitted or substituted with similar nutrient-rich alternatives. For those with a sensitivity to honey, it can be replaced with agave syrup or simply left out to reduce sweetness.

Castor Oil and Cucumber Detox Water

Beneficial effects

The Castor Oil and Cucumber Detox Water is a refreshing and hydrating blend designed to support the body's natural detoxification processes. Cucumber, with its high water content and antioxidants, aids in flushing out toxins and promotes hydration. Castor oil enhances this effect by supporting lymphatic drainage and helping to cleanse the body. This detox water is perfect for those looking to refresh their system, improve skin health, and boost overall wellness.

Ingredients

- 2 tablespoons of cold-pressed castor oil
- 1 medium cucumber, thinly sliced
- 1 gallon of filtered water
- Ice cubes (optional)
- Fresh mint leaves (optional, for added flavor and digestive benefits)

Instructions

1. In a large pitcher, combine the sliced cucumber and cold-pressed castor oil.
2. Fill the pitcher with filtered water. Stir well to ensure the castor oil is evenly distributed throughout the water.
3. If desired, add ice cubes to keep the detox water chilled and refreshing.
4. For additional flavor and digestive support, add fresh mint leaves to the pitcher.
5. Allow the mixture to infuse for at least 1 hour in the refrigerator before serving. The longer it sits, the more pronounced the flavors will be.
6. Serve the detox water in glasses, ensuring to stir the mixture before pouring to distribute the castor oil.

Variations

- For a citrus twist, add slices of lemon or lime to the pitcher. Citrus fruits can enhance the detoxifying effects and provide a boost of vitamin C.
- Incorporate slices of ginger for an extra kick and to promote healthy digestion.

Storage tips

Store the detox water in the refrigerator and consume within 24 hours for optimal freshness and efficacy. Ensure the pitcher is covered to maintain the quality and flavor of the detox water.

Tips for allergens

For those with sensitivities to cucumbers or mint, these ingredients can be omitted or substituted with other fruits or herbs, such as strawberries or basil, to suit your preferences and avoid any allergic reactions.

Castor Oil and Mint Detox Infusion

Beneficial effects

The Castor Oil and Mint Detox Infusion is designed to cleanse the body, stimulate the digestive system, and refresh the senses. Castor oil, with its detoxifying properties, aids in removing toxins from the body, while mint provides a cooling and soothing effect, helping to ease indigestion and soothe stomach discomfort. This infusion is an excellent choice for those looking to support their body's natural detoxification processes and improve overall digestive health.

Ingredients

- 2 tablespoons of cold-pressed castor oil
- 1 cup of fresh mint leaves
- 1 tablespoon of lemon juice
- 1 teaspoon of honey (optional, for sweetness)
- 2 cups of boiling water

Instructions

1. Place the fresh mint leaves in a large mug or heat-proof container.
2. Pour the boiling water over the mint leaves and allow them to steep for about 10 minutes.
3. Strain the mint leaves from the water and discard them.
4. Stir in the cold-pressed castor oil and lemon juice into the mint-infused water until well combined.
5. If desired, add honey to taste and mix thoroughly.
6. Consume the detox infusion warm, preferably in the morning on an empty stomach, to maximize its cleansing effects.

Variations

- For an extra detox boost, add a slice of ginger to the infusion while the mint leaves are steeping. Ginger has additional anti-inflammatory and digestive benefits.
- If you prefer a cold beverage, allow the infusion to cool to room temperature, then refrigerate for 1-2 hours. Serve over ice for a refreshing detox drink.

Storage tips

It's best to prepare the Castor Oil and Mint Detox Infusion fresh for each use to ensure the potency of the ingredients. However, if you need to prepare it in advance, store the mint-infused water (without the castor oil and lemon juice) in the refrigerator for up to 24 hours. Add the castor oil and lemon juice just before consumption.

Tips for allergens

If you are allergic to honey, you can omit it from the recipe or substitute it with maple syrup. Always ensure that you are not allergic to any of the ingredients by performing a patch test or consulting with a healthcare provider before incorporating this detox infusion into your routine.

Castor Oil and Pineapple Detox Shake

Beneficial effects

The Castor Oil and Pineapple Detox Shake is a refreshing and powerful detoxifying blend designed to cleanse the body, boost digestion, and promote weight loss. Castor oil's laxative properties aid in the removal of toxins from the digestive system, while pineapple, rich in bromelain, supports digestion, reduces inflammation, and enhances the body's detoxification processes. This shake also provides a healthy dose of vitamins, minerals, and antioxidants, contributing to overall wellness and vitality.

Ingredients

- 1 tablespoon of cold-pressed castor oil
- 1 cup of fresh pineapple chunks
- 1 cup of coconut water or filtered water
- 1/2 banana (for sweetness and texture)
- A handful of spinach (optional, for added nutrients)
- Ice cubes (optional, for a chilled shake)

Instructions

1. Place the fresh pineapple chunks, banana, and spinach (if using) into a blender.
2. Add the cold-pressed castor oil and coconut water or filtered water to the blender.
3. Blend the mixture on high until smooth and creamy.
4. Add ice cubes to the blender (if desired) and blend again until the shake reaches your preferred consistency.
5. Pour the shake into a glass and enjoy immediately for the best detoxifying benefits.

Variations

- For an extra boost of protein, add a scoop of your favorite plant-based protein powder to the shake.
- If you prefer a sweeter shake, include a tablespoon of honey or maple syrup.
- To increase the detoxifying effects, add a teaspoon of ground flaxseed or chia seeds for added fiber.

Storage tips

Due to the fresh ingredients and the inclusion of castor oil, it's best to consume the detox shake immediately after preparation. If needed, the shake can be stored in the refrigerator for up to 2 hours, but shake well before consuming as the ingredients may separate over time.

Tips for allergens

If you are allergic to bananas, you can substitute it with avocado to maintain the creamy texture without compromising the taste. For those with sensitivities to pineapple, mango can be a suitable alternative, offering similar digestive benefits.

Castor Oil and Beetroot Detox Blend

Beneficial effects
The Castor Oil and Beetroot Detox Blend is a potent detoxifying drink designed to cleanse the liver and blood, improve digestion, and boost the immune system. Castor oil's lymphatic-supportive properties help in the detoxification process, while beetroot is rich in antioxidants, vitamins, and minerals that purify the blood and support liver health. This blend is ideal for those looking to naturally detoxify their body and enhance overall wellness.

Ingredients
- 2 tablespoons of cold-pressed castor oil
- 1 medium beetroot, peeled and chopped
- 1 cup of water
- Juice of 1/2 lemon
- 1 tablespoon of honey (optional, for sweetness)

Instructions
1. Place the chopped beetroot and water in a blender and blend until smooth.
2. Strain the beetroot juice into a glass to remove any pulp.
3. Add the cold-pressed castor oil and lemon juice to the beetroot juice. Stir well to combine.
4. If desired, add honey to the mixture for added sweetness and mix thoroughly.
5. Consume the detox blend first thing in the morning on an empty stomach to maximize its cleansing effects.

Variations
- For an additional detox boost, add a pinch of ground turmeric or ginger to the blend. Both spices have anti-inflammatory properties and can enhance the detoxification process.
- If you prefer a thinner consistency, add an extra 1/2 cup of water to the mixture.

Storage tips
It's best to prepare this detox blend fresh each morning to ensure the potency of the nutrients. However, if you need to prepare it in advance, store the mixture in the refrigerator for no more than 24 hours in a sealed glass container.

Tips for allergens
If you are allergic to beets, you can substitute them with carrots, which also have detoxifying properties and a high nutrient content. For those sensitive to honey, it can be omitted or replaced with maple syrup as a natural sweetener.

Mental Wellness Remedies

Castor Oil and Lavender Stress Relief Balm

Beneficial effects
The Castor Oil and Lavender Stress Relief Balm is a soothing and therapeutic remedy designed to alleviate stress, promote relaxation, and enhance mental wellness. The combination of castor oil and lavender essential oil creates a powerful blend that not only calms the mind but also moisturizes the skin, making it a perfect solution for those seeking a natural way to manage stress and anxiety.

Ingredients
- 2 tablespoons of cold-pressed castor oil
- 2 tablespoons of coconut oil
- 2 tablespoons of beeswax pellets
- 10-15 drops of lavender essential oil
- Small glass jar for storage

Instructions
1. In a double boiler, melt the coconut oil and beeswax pellets together over low heat until fully dissolved.
2. Remove from heat and allow the mixture to cool slightly before adding the cold-pressed castor oil. Stir well to ensure all ingredients are evenly combined.
3. Add the lavender essential oil to the mixture and stir again to distribute the oil throughout the balm.
4. Carefully pour the balm into the small glass jar and allow it to cool and solidify at room temperature.
5. Once solidified, seal the jar. Your stress relief balm is ready for use.

Variations
- For those sensitive to lavender, chamomile essential oil can be used as a gentle alternative that also provides calming and soothing properties.
- Add a few drops of vitamin E oil to the mixture for added skin nourishment and antioxidant benefits.

Storage tips
Store the balm in a cool, dark place to maintain its potency and freshness. Ensure the jar is tightly sealed to prevent the balm from drying out. When stored properly, the balm should remain effective for up to 6 months.

Tips for allergens
If you have a sensitivity or allergy to coconut oil, it can be substituted with shea butter for a similar consistency and moisturizing properties. Always perform a patch test on a small area of your skin before applying the balm extensively, especially if incorporating new ingredients into your regimen.

Castor Oil and Chamomile Calming Tea

Beneficial effects

The Castor Oil and Chamomile Calming Tea is a soothing beverage designed to promote mental wellness by reducing stress and anxiety levels. Castor oil, with its anti-inflammatory properties, aids in soothing the nervous system, while chamomile is widely recognized for its calming and relaxing effects. This tea is perfect for unwinding after a stressful day, promoting a sense of calm, and preparing the body and mind for a restful night's sleep.

Ingredients

- 2 tablespoons of cold-pressed castor oil
- 1 chamomile tea bag or 1 tablespoon of dried chamomile flowers
- 1 cup of boiling water
- Honey or lemon to taste (optional)

Instructions

1. Place the chamomile tea bag or dried chamomile flowers in a cup.
2. Pour the boiling water over the chamomile and allow it to steep for 5-10 minutes.
3. Remove the tea bag or strain the tea to remove the flowers.
4. Stir in the cold-pressed castor oil until it is well integrated into the tea.
5. If desired, add honey or lemon to taste, and stir well.
6. Enjoy the tea warm, ideally before bedtime, to maximize its calming effects.

Variations

- For added relaxation, include a few drops of lavender essential oil to the tea after steeping. Lavender enhances the calming properties of chamomile.
- If you prefer a caffeine-free boost of energy, add a slice of fresh ginger to the tea while it steeps. Ginger can invigorate the senses without disrupting relaxation.

Storage tips

It's best to prepare the Castor Oil and Chamomile Calming Tea fresh for each use to ensure the effectiveness of the ingredients. However, chamomile tea (without castor oil) can be made in advance and stored in the refrigerator for up to 48 hours. Add castor oil to individual servings as needed.

Tips for allergens

If you have allergies to chamomile, consider substituting it with green tea for its calming amino acid, L-theanine. For those sensitive to honey, it can be omitted or replaced with maple syrup as a natural sweetener.

Castor Oil and Peppermint Headache Relief

Beneficial effects

The Castor Oil and Peppermint Headache Relief is a natural remedy designed to alleviate tension headaches and migraines. Castor oil, with its anti-inflammatory properties, helps to soothe pain and reduce swelling, while peppermint oil provides a cooling sensation that can relieve the discomfort associated with headaches. This combination is effective for those seeking a quick and natural solution to headache pain.

Ingredients

- 2 tablespoons of cold-pressed castor oil
- 5 drops of peppermint essential oil
- A clean, soft cloth or cotton pad

Instructions

1. In a small bowl, mix the cold-pressed castor oil with the peppermint essential oil until well combined.
2. Soak the clean, soft cloth or cotton pad in the oil mixture, making sure it is fully saturated.
3. Gently apply the soaked cloth or cotton pad to the forehead or temples, wherever the headache pain is most intense.
4. Leave the cloth or cotton pad in place for 15-20 minutes, lying down in a comfortable position if possible.
5. Remove the cloth or cotton pad and wash the area with cool water.

Variations

- For additional relaxation and enhanced pain relief, add 2 drops of lavender essential oil to the mixture. Lavender's calming properties can help reduce stress, a common trigger for headaches.
- If the sensation of peppermint is too intense, dilute the mixture with an additional tablespoon of castor oil.

Storage tips

Prepare the mixture fresh for each use to ensure the essential oils retain their potency. Any leftover castor oil can be stored in a cool, dark place for future use.

Tips for allergens

If you are sensitive to peppermint or lavender essential oil, test the mixture on a small patch of skin before applying it to your forehead or temples. Adjust the essential oil concentration as needed to avoid irritation.

Castor Oil and Lemon Balm Sleep Aid

Beneficial effects

The Castor Oil and Lemon Balm Sleep Aid is a natural remedy designed to promote relaxation, ease anxiety, and support a restful night's sleep. Castor oil, with its anti-inflammatory properties, can help soothe tension and discomfort that may hinder sleep, while lemon balm is known for its calming effects on the mind and body, reducing stress and improving sleep quality.

Ingredients

-   2 tablespoons of cold-pressed castor oil
-   1 tablespoon of dried lemon balm leaves
-   1 cup of boiling water
-   Honey to taste (optional)

Instructions

1. Place dried lemon balm leaves in a cup or teapot.
2. Pour boiling water over the lemon balm leaves and allow to steep for 10 minutes.
3. Strain the lemon balm tea into a mug, removing the leaves.
4. Stir in the cold-pressed castor oil until it is well combined with the tea.
5. Add honey to taste, if desired, and stir well.
6. Drink the sleep aid about 30 minutes before bedtime to allow the body to relax and prepare for sleep.

Variations

-   For additional relaxation benefits, add a few drops of lavender essential oil to the mixture. Lavender's soothing scent enhances the calming effects of the sleep aid.
-   If you prefer a cold beverage, allow the tea to cool to room temperature before adding the castor oil and honey. You can also refrigerate it for a refreshing night-time drink.

Storage tips

It's best to prepare the Castor Oil and Lemon Balm Sleep Aid fresh each evening to ensure the potency and effectiveness of the ingredients. However, the lemon balm tea (without the castor oil and honey) can be prepared in advance and stored in the refrigerator for up to 24 hours. Add the castor oil and honey just before consumption.

Tips for allergens

If you are allergic to lemon balm or honey, you can omit these ingredients. Lemon balm can be substituted with chamomile, which also has sleep-promoting properties. For those who cannot consume honey, consider using maple syrup as a sweetener or simply enjoy the tea without any added sweeteners.

Castor Oil and Valerian Root Relaxation Tonic

Beneficial effects
The Castor Oil and Valerian Root Relaxation Tonic is a natural remedy designed to alleviate stress, promote relaxation, and improve sleep quality. Castor oil's anti-inflammatory properties help to soothe the nervous system, while valerian root is widely recognized for its sedative qualities that can ease anxiety and foster a sense of calm. This tonic is particularly beneficial for individuals experiencing stress, insomnia, or restlessness, offering a holistic approach to mental wellness.

Ingredients
- 2 tablespoons of cold-pressed castor oil
- 1 teaspoon of dried valerian root
- 1 cup of boiling water
- Honey or lemon to taste (optional)

Instructions
1. Place the dried valerian root in a cup or teapot.
2. Pour the boiling water over the valerian root and cover. Allow it to steep for 10-15 minutes to extract the beneficial properties of the herb.
3. Strain the valerian root from the water and let the tea cool to a comfortable temperature.
4. Stir in the cold-pressed castor oil into the valerian tea until well combined.
5. Add honey or lemon to taste, if desired, and stir again.
6. Consume this tonic 30 minutes before bedtime to promote relaxation and improve sleep quality.

Variations
- For an added calming effect, include a few drops of lavender essential oil to the tonic. Lavender's soothing scent enhances the relaxation benefits.
- If you prefer a cold beverage, allow the tonic to cool completely and refrigerate for 1-2 hours before consuming. Serve over ice for a refreshing, calming drink.

Storage tips
Prepare the Castor Oil and Valerian Root Relaxation Tonic fresh each evening to ensure the effectiveness of the valerian root. It is not recommended to store any prepared tonic as the potency of the ingredients is best when fresh.

Tips for allergens
If you are allergic to valerian root, consider substituting it with chamomile, which also has calming properties. For those with sensitivities to honey or lemon, these ingredients can be omitted without affecting the tonic's relaxation benefits.

Castor Oil and Passionflower Anxiety Relief

Beneficial effects

The Castor Oil and Passionflower Anxiety Relief blend is a natural remedy designed to alleviate symptoms of anxiety, promote relaxation, and improve sleep quality. Castor oil, known for its soothing properties, works in harmony with passionflower, a herb celebrated for its efficacy in reducing nervous tension and treating anxiety. This combination offers a gentle yet effective approach to managing stress and anxiety, providing a sense of calm and well-being.

Ingredients

- 2 tablespoons of cold-pressed castor oil
- 1 tablespoon of dried passionflower
- 1 cup of boiling water
- Honey or lemon to taste (optional)

Instructions

1. Place the dried passionflower in a heat-proof container or teapot.
2. Pour the boiling water over the passionflower and cover. Allow it to steep for 10-15 minutes to extract the beneficial compounds.
3. Strain the passionflower tea into a mug, removing the dried herb.
4. Stir in the cold-pressed castor oil until it is well integrated into the tea.
5. If desired, add honey or lemon to taste, and stir well.
6. Consume this blend in the evening, about 30 minutes before bedtime, to promote relaxation and support restful sleep.

Variations

- For added calming effects, include a few drops of lavender essential oil into the tea after adding the castor oil. Lavender enhances the anxiety-relieving properties and adds a pleasant aroma.
- If you prefer a cold beverage, allow the tea to cool to room temperature before adding the castor oil and refrigerate for 1-2 hours. Serve over ice for a refreshing anxiety-relieving drink.

Storage tips

Prepare the Castor Oil and Passionflower Anxiety Relief blend fresh for each use to ensure the effectiveness of the ingredients. However, the passionflower tea (without castor oil) can be made in advance and stored in the refrigerator for up to 24 hours. Add castor oil and optional ingredients just before consumption.

Tips for allergens

If you are allergic to passionflower, you can substitute it with chamomile, which also has calming and anxiety-relieving properties. For those sensitive to honey, it can be omitted or replaced with a sweetener of your choice. Always consult with a healthcare provider before starting any new herbal remedy, especially if you have existing health conditions or are taking medications.

Castor Oil and Ashwagandha Mood Booster

Beneficial effects

The Castor Oil and Ashwagandha Mood Booster is a natural remedy designed to alleviate stress, reduce anxiety, and improve overall mood. Castor oil, with its soothing properties, works to calm the nervous system, while ashwagandha is known for its ability to combat stress, enhance stamina, and promote mental clarity. This combination makes the mood booster an excellent choice for those seeking a natural way to maintain emotional balance and enhance well-being.

Ingredients

- 2 tablespoons of cold-pressed castor oil
- 1 teaspoon of ashwagandha powder
- 1 cup of warm milk (dairy or plant-based)
- Honey to taste (optional)

Instructions

1. Warm the milk in a saucepan over low heat until it is just warm to the touch.
2. Add the ashwagandha powder to the warm milk and stir well to ensure it is fully dissolved.
3. Stir in the cold-pressed castor oil, mixing thoroughly to combine with the ashwagandha-infused milk.
4. If desired, add honey to taste for sweetness.
5. Consume this mood-boosting beverage in the evening, about 30 minutes before bedtime, to promote relaxation and a restful night's sleep.

Variations

- For a vegan version, use almond, coconut, or oat milk as a plant-based alternative to dairy milk.
- To enhance the calming effects, add a pinch of cinnamon or turmeric to the mixture. Both spices offer additional anti-inflammatory benefits and can improve the flavor of the drink.

Storage tips

Prepare the Castor Oil and Ashwagandha Mood Booster fresh each time to ensure the potency of the ingredients. It is not recommended to store any prepared mixture as the natural properties are best when consumed immediately after preparation.

Tips for allergens

If you are allergic to dairy, opt for a plant-based milk alternative. Always ensure that you are not allergic to ashwagandha by performing a patch test or consulting with a healthcare provider before incorporating it into your routine.

Castor Oil and Holy Basil Stress Reducer

Beneficial effects

The Castor Oil and Holy Basil Stress Reducer is a natural remedy designed to alleviate stress, reduce anxiety, and promote a sense of calm and well-being. Castor oil, with its soothing properties, combined with the adaptogenic benefits of holy basil (Tulsi), helps to balance the stress hormones in the body, offering relief from the physical and mental effects of stress. This remedy is particularly beneficial for those seeking a natural approach to managing stress, improving mood, and enhancing overall mental wellness.

Ingredients

- 2 tablespoons of cold-pressed castor oil
- 1 tablespoon of dried holy basil leaves
- 1 cup of boiling water
- Honey or lemon to taste (optional)

Instructions

1. Place the dried holy basil leaves in a heat-proof container or teapot.
2. Pour the boiling water over the holy basil leaves and cover. Allow it to steep for 10-15 minutes to create a strong infusion.
3. Strain the holy basil leaves from the water and discard them.
4. Stir in the cold-pressed castor oil into the holy basil tea until well combined.
5. If desired, add honey or lemon to taste, and mix thoroughly.
6. Consume this stress-reducing tonic once daily, preferably in the evening, to promote relaxation and stress relief.

Variations

- For added relaxation benefits, include a teaspoon of lavender flowers to the infusion. Lavender is known for its calming effects on the nervous system.
- If you prefer a cold beverage, allow the tonic to cool to room temperature, then refrigerate for 1-2 hours. Serve over ice for a refreshing stress-relief drink.

Storage tips

Prepare the Castor Oil and Holy Basil Stress Reducer fresh each time to ensure the maximum therapeutic benefits of the ingredients. However, the holy basil tea (without castor oil) can be prepared in advance and stored in the refrigerator for up to 48 hours. Add castor oil to individual servings as needed.

Tips for allergens

If you are allergic to holy basil, you can substitute it with chamomile, which also offers stress-reducing properties. For those with sensitivities to honey, it can be omitted or replaced with a natural sweetener of your choice.

Castor Oil and Rhodiola Energy Enhancer

Beneficial effects

The Castor Oil and Rhodiola Energy Enhancer is formulated to boost energy levels, improve mental clarity, and support the body's stress response. Castor oil's anti-inflammatory properties help in soothing the nervous system, while Rhodiola, an adaptogen, enhances stamina, reduces fatigue, and helps the body adapt to stress more effectively. This combination is ideal for those experiencing low energy, mental fog, or the physical effects of stress.

Ingredients

- 2 tablespoons of cold-pressed castor oil
- 1 teaspoon of Rhodiola rosea extract
- 1 cup of warm water
- Honey to taste (optional)

Instructions

1. Warm the water to a comfortable drinking temperature.
2. Add the Rhodiola rosea extract and cold-pressed castor oil to the warm water. Stir thoroughly until both are well combined.
3. If desired, add honey to taste for sweetness, and mix well.
4. Consume this energy enhancer in the morning, preferably on an empty stomach, to kickstart your day with increased vitality and mental clarity.

Variations

- For an added flavor and antioxidant boost, include a squeeze of fresh lemon juice.
- If you prefer a cooler beverage, let the mixture cool to room temperature, then add ice cubes for a refreshing energy drink.

Storage tips

Prepare the Castor Oil and Rhodiola Energy Enhancer fresh each morning to ensure the effectiveness of the ingredients. It is not recommended to store any prepared mixture as the active properties are best when fresh.

Tips for allergens

If you are sensitive to honey, you can omit it from the recipe or substitute it with maple syrup. Always ensure that you are not allergic to Rhodiola rosea by performing a patch test or consulting with a healthcare provider before incorporating this enhancer into your routine.

Castor Oil and Ginkgo Biloba Memory Support

Beneficial effects

The Castor Oil and Ginkgo Biloba Memory Support concoction is designed to enhance cognitive function, improve memory retention, and support overall brain health. Castor oil, known for its anti-inflammatory properties, aids in promoting healthy blood flow to the brain, while Ginkgo Biloba is renowned for its ability to improve cognitive performance and protect neural health. This combination makes for a potent natural remedy to support memory, focus, and protect against cognitive decline.

Ingredients

-   2 tablespoons of cold-pressed castor oil
-   1 teaspoon of Ginkgo Biloba extract
-   1 cup of warm water
-   Honey or lemon to taste (optional)

Instructions

1. Warm the water to a comfortable drinking temperature.
2. Add the Ginkgo Biloba extract to the warm water and stir well.
3. Incorporate the cold-pressed castor oil into the Ginkgo Biloba mixture, ensuring it's fully mixed.
4. If desired, add honey or lemon to taste, and stir until dissolved.
5. Consume this mixture once daily, preferably in the morning, to support cognitive function and memory.

Variations

-   For those looking to enhance the brain-boosting effects, adding a pinch of turmeric to the mixture can provide additional anti-inflammatory and antioxidant benefits.
-   If the taste of castor oil is too strong, you can mix the concoction with a small amount of natural fruit juice to improve palatability.

Storage tips

Prepare the Castor Oil and Ginkgo Biloba Memory Support mixture fresh each time to ensure the effectiveness of the ingredients. It is not recommended to store the prepared mixture due to the potential degradation of active compounds.

Tips for allergens

If you are sensitive to Ginkgo Biloba or castor oil, start with a smaller dose to assess tolerance. Consult with a healthcare provider before incorporating this remedy into your routine, especially if you have existing health conditions or are taking medication.

Women's Health Recipes

Castor Oil and Red Raspberry Leaf Menstrual Relief Tea

Beneficial effects
The Castor Oil and Red Raspberry Leaf Menstrual Relief Tea is a natural remedy designed to alleviate menstrual discomfort, reduce cramping, and balance hormones. Castor oil's anti-inflammatory properties help soothe the reproductive organs, while red raspberry leaf is traditionally used to tone the uterus and ease menstrual pain. This tea offers a gentle, effective way to manage symptoms associated with menstruation, promoting a more comfortable menstrual cycle.

Ingredients
- 2 tablespoons of cold-pressed castor oil
- 1 tablespoon of dried red raspberry leaves
- 1 cup of boiling water
- Honey or lemon to taste (optional)

Instructions
1. Place the dried red raspberry leaves in a cup or teapot.
2. Pour the boiling water over the leaves and allow them to steep for 10-15 minutes.
3. Strain the tea into a mug, removing the leaves.
4. Stir in the cold-pressed castor oil until it is well integrated into the tea.
5. Add honey or lemon to taste, if desired, and stir well.
6. Consume one cup of the tea daily, starting a few days before the onset of menstruation and continuing through the first few days of your cycle.

Variations
- For additional hormonal support, include a teaspoon of dried chaste berry (Vitex) with the red raspberry leaves while steeping.
- If experiencing heavy menstrual flow, add a pinch of cinnamon to the tea for its natural astringent properties.

Storage tips
Prepare the Castor Oil and Red Raspberry Leaf Menstrual Relief Tea fresh for each use to ensure the maximum therapeutic benefits. However, you can store extra dried red raspberry leaves in a cool, dry place, away from direct sunlight, to maintain their potency for future use.

Tips for allergens
If you are sensitive to honey, you can substitute it with maple syrup or simply enjoy the tea without any sweeteners. Always ensure that you are not allergic to red raspberry leaves by performing a patch test or consulting with a healthcare provider before incorporating this tea into your routine.

Castor Oil and Dong Quai Hormone Balance Tonic

Beneficial effects

The Castor Oil and Dong Quai Hormone Balance Tonic is specifically formulated to support hormonal balance, alleviate menstrual discomfort, and enhance reproductive health. Castor oil's anti-inflammatory properties help soothe the reproductive organs, while Dong Quai, known as the "female ginseng," naturally balances estrogen levels, improves circulation to the reproductive system, and relieves symptoms of menopause and PMS.

Ingredients

- 2 tablespoons of cold-pressed castor oil
- 1 teaspoon of Dong Quai extract
- 1 cup of warm water
- Honey or lemon to taste (optional)

Instructions

1. Warm the water to a comfortable drinking temperature.
2. Add the Dong Quai extract to the warm water and stir well.
3. Stir in the cold-pressed castor oil, ensuring it's fully mixed with the Dong Quai-infused water.
4. Add honey or lemon to taste, if desired, and mix thoroughly.
5. Consume this tonic once daily, preferably in the morning, to promote hormonal balance and alleviate menstrual discomfort.

Variations

- For added benefits, include a pinch of ground cinnamon or ginger to the tonic. Both spices can enhance circulation and provide additional relief from menstrual cramps.
- If you prefer a cooler beverage, allow the tonic to cool to room temperature before adding the castor oil and then refrigerate for 1-2 hours. Serve chilled.

Storage tips

It's best to prepare the Castor Oil and Dong Quai Hormone Balance Tonic fresh each morning to ensure the effectiveness of the ingredients. However, the Dong Quai-infused water (without castor oil) can be prepared in advance and stored in the refrigerator for up to 48 hours. Add castor oil to individual servings as needed.

Tips for allergens

If you are allergic to Dong Quai, consider consulting with a healthcare provider for alternative herbal options that support hormonal balance. For those sensitive to honey, it can be omitted or replaced with a natural sweetener of your choice.

Castor Oil and Black Cohosh Menopause Support Serum

Beneficial effects

The Castor Oil and Black Cohosh Menopause Support Serum is specifically formulated to provide relief from menopausal symptoms such as hot flashes, mood swings, and hormonal imbalances. Castor oil, with its anti-inflammatory and moisturizing properties, helps to soothe skin irritation and maintain skin health, while black cohosh is known for its ability to mimic estrogen in the body, offering natural relief from menopause-related discomforts. This serum aims to balance hormones naturally, promote emotional well-being, and support overall women's health during menopause.

Ingredients

-   3 tablespoons of cold-pressed castor oil
-   1 tablespoon of black cohosh extract
-   1/4 cup of almond oil (as a carrier oil)
-   5 drops of lavender essential oil (for additional calming effects)
-   Small glass bottle with dropper

Instructions

1. In a clean bowl, mix the cold-pressed castor oil with the almond oil thoroughly. Almond oil is used as a carrier to dilute the potent black cohosh extract and facilitate application.
2. Add the black cohosh extract to the oil mixture and stir well to ensure all ingredients are evenly blended.
3. Incorporate the lavender essential oil into the serum for its calming and soothing properties.
4. Using a funnel, carefully transfer the serum into the glass dropper bottle.
5. To use, apply 2-3 drops of the serum to the palms of your hands and gently massage into the skin on your neck, chest, or any area affected by menopausal symptoms. Use once daily, preferably at night before bed.

Variations

-   For those with sensitive skin, you can substitute almond oil with jojoba oil, which is lighter and less likely to cause irritation.
-   If you prefer a fragrance-free option, omit the lavender essential oil from the recipe.

Storage tips

Store the menopause support serum in a cool, dark place to preserve the potency of the ingredients. Ensure the dropper bottle is tightly sealed to prevent oxidation. When stored properly, the serum should remain effective for up to 6 months.

Tips for allergens

If you are allergic to almond oil, substituting it with coconut oil or olive oil can provide similar benefits without the risk of an allergic reaction. Always perform a patch test on a small area of your skin before using the serum extensively, especially if you're incorporating new ingredients into your regimen.

Castor Oil and Evening Primrose Oil PMS Relief Balm

Beneficial effects
The Castor Oil and Evening Primrose Oil PMS Relief Balm is specially formulated to alleviate symptoms of premenstrual syndrome (PMS), including cramps, mood swings, and breast tenderness. Castor oil, known for its anti-inflammatory and analgesic properties, helps to soothe cramps and reduce discomfort, while evening primrose oil, rich in gamma-linolenic acid (GLA), aids in balancing hormonal fluctuations that contribute to PMS symptoms. This balm provides a natural, therapeutic way to manage PMS, promoting a sense of calm and well-being during the menstrual cycle.

Ingredients
- 2 tablespoons of cold-pressed castor oil
- 2 tablespoons of evening primrose oil
- 1/4 cup of coconut oil
- 2 tablespoons of beeswax pellets
- 10 drops of lavender essential oil (optional for additional calming effects)

Instructions
1. In a double boiler, melt the beeswax pellets over low heat until completely liquid.
2. Add the coconut oil to the melted beeswax and stir until the two are well combined and fully melted together.
3. Remove the mixture from heat and allow it to cool slightly before adding the castor oil and evening primrose oil. Stir well to ensure all oils are evenly integrated.
4. If using, incorporate the lavender essential oil into the mixture for its calming and soothing properties.
5. Pour the balm into a clean, dry container and allow it to cool and solidify at room temperature.
6. Once solidified, seal the container. The PMS relief balm is now ready for use.

Variations
- For those sensitive to lavender, chamomile essential oil can be used as a gentle alternative that also provides calming and anti-inflammatory benefits.
- To create a softer balm, reduce the amount of beeswax to 1 tablespoon. This adjustment is particularly beneficial if you prefer a balm that is easier to apply.

Storage tips
Store the PMS relief balm in a cool, dry place, away from direct sunlight. Ensure the container is tightly sealed to maintain the balm's potency and prevent it from drying out. When stored properly, the balm should remain effective for up to 6 months.

Tips for allergens
If you have a sensitivity or allergy to any of the essential oils, you can omit them from the recipe. Always perform a patch test on a small area of your skin before applying the balm extensively, especially if incorporating new ingredients into your regimen.

Castor Oil and Chasteberry Fertility Boost Elixir

Beneficial effects

The Castor Oil and Chasteberry Fertility Boost Elixir is designed to support reproductive health and enhance fertility naturally. Castor oil, with its ability to improve circulation and promote healing within the body, works alongside chasteberry, a herb known for its efficacy in balancing hormones, particularly progesterone, which is crucial for maintaining pregnancy. This elixir can help regulate menstrual cycles, alleviate symptoms of PMS, and increase the likelihood of conception for those trying to conceive.

Ingredients

- 2 tablespoons of cold-pressed castor oil
- 1 teaspoon of dried chasteberry (Vitex)
- 1 cup of hot water
- Honey to taste (optional)

Instructions

1. Steep the dried chasteberry in hot water for 10-15 minutes to make a strong tea.
2. Strain the chasteberry, ensuring to press out all the liquid from the herbs.
3. Allow the tea to cool to a comfortable drinking temperature.
4. Stir in the cold-pressed castor oil until it is well combined with the chasteberry tea.
5. Add honey to taste, if desired, and mix thoroughly.
6. Consume one cup of the elixir daily, preferably in the morning on an empty stomach, to support fertility and hormonal balance.

Variations

- For those who prefer a cold beverage, allow the elixir to cool completely and then refrigerate. Serve chilled.
- To enhance the flavor and add additional health benefits, include a squeeze of fresh lemon juice, which can also aid in detoxification.

Storage tips

It is best to prepare the Castor Oil and Chasteberry Fertility Boost Elixir fresh each day to ensure the potency of the ingredients. However, the chasteberry tea can be made in advance and stored in the refrigerator for up to 48 hours. Add castor oil and optional honey just before consumption.

Tips for allergens

If you are allergic to chasteberry or have a sensitivity to hormone-related herbs, consult with a healthcare provider before starting this regimen. Honey can be omitted for those with allergies or substituted with a different natural sweetener like maple syrup.

Castor Oil and Fenugreek Breast Health Massage Oil

Beneficial effects

The Castor Oil and Fenugreek Breast Health Massage Oil is specifically formulated to support breast health, promote lymphatic drainage, and potentially assist in enhancing the firmness of breast tissue. Castor oil, known for its anti-inflammatory and lymphatic stimulant properties, works in tandem with fenugreek, which is traditionally used for its benefits in women's health, including its potential to naturally increase breast size and promote overall breast health.

Ingredients

- 2 tablespoons of cold-pressed castor oil
- 1 tablespoon of fenugreek seed powder
- 1/2 cup of almond oil (as a carrier oil)
- 5 drops of lavender essential oil (optional for additional soothing effects and aroma)

Instructions

1. In a clean bowl, mix the fenugreek seed powder with the almond oil until the powder is fully dissolved.
2. Add the cold-pressed castor oil to the mixture and stir well to ensure all ingredients are thoroughly combined.
3. If using, incorporate the lavender essential oil into the blend for its calming scent and additional skin-soothing benefits.
4. Transfer the massage oil into a clean, dark glass bottle to preserve the integrity of the oils.
5. To use, gently massage a small amount of the oil onto the breast area in circular motions, focusing on the outward areas and moving towards the armpits to promote lymphatic drainage. Avoid direct contact with the nipples.
6. Perform the massage 2-3 times a week, preferably after a warm shower when the skin is still slightly damp to enhance absorption.

Variations

- For a warming effect, which can further promote circulation, add 2 drops of ginger essential oil to the mixture.
- If almond oil is not available or if you're allergic, jojoba oil can be used as a substitute carrier oil with similar moisturizing properties.

Storage tips

Store the breast health massage oil in a cool, dark place, away from direct sunlight. The dark glass bottle will help protect the oils from light degradation, ensuring the mixture remains potent for up to 6 months.

Tips for allergens

If you have sensitive skin or are allergic to any of the ingredients listed, perform a patch test on a small area of your skin before applying the oil extensively. Substitute fenugreek seed powder with flaxseed oil for similar health benefits if fenugreek is not suitable for your skin type.

Castor Oil and Sage Hot Flash Relief Spray

Beneficial effects

The Castor Oil and Sage Hot Flash Relief Spray offers a natural and effective solution for managing hot flashes and night sweats associated with menopause. Castor oil, with its cooling and anti-inflammatory properties, helps to soothe the skin and regulate temperature, while sage is renowned for its ability to reduce perspiration and balance hormone levels. This spray provides immediate relief from discomfort, promoting a sense of calm and comfort during menopausal transitions.

Ingredients

- 2 tablespoons of cold-pressed castor oil
- 1/4 cup of distilled water
- 1/4 cup of sage leaves or 10 drops of sage essential oil
- 1 tablespoon of witch hazel (optional, for added cooling effect)
- Small spray bottle

Instructions

1. If using sage leaves, begin by boiling the distilled water and pouring it over the sage leaves. Allow the mixture to steep for 30 minutes to create a sage infusion. Strain the leaves from the water and let the infusion cool to room temperature.
2. Combine the sage infusion or sage essential oil with cold-pressed castor oil in a bowl. Mix thoroughly to ensure the ingredients are well blended.
3. Add witch hazel to the mixture if using, and stir well. Witch hazel enhances the cooling and soothing properties of the spray.
4. Using a funnel, carefully pour the mixture into the small spray bottle.
5. To use, shake the bottle well and spray directly onto the skin whenever hot flashes or night sweats occur. Allow it to air dry for the best cooling effect.

Variations

- For a more potent spray, increase the amount of sage essential oil to 15 drops.
- Add a few drops of peppermint essential oil for an extra cooling sensation and refreshing scent.

Storage tips

Store the hot flash relief spray in a cool, dark place, preferably in the refrigerator for an enhanced cooling effect upon application. Ensure the spray bottle is tightly sealed to preserve the potency of the ingredients. Use within 1 month for optimal effectiveness.

Tips for allergens

If you are sensitive to sage or witch hazel, you can omit these ingredients and substitute the sage with lavender or chamomile, which also have soothing properties. Always perform a patch test on a small area of your skin before using the spray extensively, especially if incorporating new ingredients into your regimen.

Castor Oil and Nettle Leaf Iron Boost Tonic

Beneficial effects

The Castor Oil and Nettle Leaf Iron Boost Tonic is a natural remedy aimed at improving iron levels and enhancing overall blood health. Castor oil, with its ability to support lymphatic circulation, combined with nettle leaf, rich in iron and vitamins, works synergistically to increase iron absorption and stimulate the production of red blood cells. This tonic is especially beneficial for individuals experiencing fatigue, weakness, or anemia due to low iron levels, offering a holistic approach to restoring vitality and energy.

Ingredients

- 2 tablespoons of cold-pressed castor oil
- 1 cup of fresh nettle leaves or 2 tablespoons of dried nettle leaves
- 2 cups of water
- Juice of 1 lemon (for vitamin C to enhance iron absorption)
- Honey to taste (optional, for sweetness)

Instructions

1. If using fresh nettle leaves, thoroughly wash them under running water. For dried nettle leaves, ensure they are free from any debris.
2. In a medium saucepan, bring the water to a boil. Add the nettle leaves to the boiling water and reduce the heat.
3. Simmer the nettle leaves for 10 minutes to create a strong infusion.
4. Strain the nettle leaves from the water and allow the nettle tea to cool to a warm, drinkable temperature.
5. Stir in the cold-pressed castor oil and lemon juice into the nettle tea. Mix thoroughly until the castor oil is well integrated.
6. Add honey to taste, if desired, and stir well.
7. Consume a cup of this tonic daily, preferably in the morning, to support iron levels and enhance blood health.

Variations

- For an added nutritional boost, blend the tonic with a handful of spinach before straining. Spinach is another excellent source of iron and vitamins.
- If you prefer a cold beverage, refrigerate the tonic for 1-2 hours and serve over ice for a refreshing drink.

Storage tips

Prepare the tonic fresh each morning for optimal benefits. However, if you need to prepare it in advance, store the nettle tea (without the castor oil and lemon juice) in the refrigerator for up to 48 hours. Add the castor oil and lemon juice just before consumption.

Tips for allergens

If you are allergic to nettle, consider substituting it with another iron-rich herb such as dandelion leaves. Always perform a patch test on your skin with diluted nettle extract to ensure there is no adverse reaction before consuming the tonic regularly.

Castor Oil and Maca Root Libido Enhancer

Beneficial effects

The Castor Oil and Maca Root Libido Enhancer is a natural remedy formulated to improve sexual health and vitality. Castor oil, known for its circulatory and anti-inflammatory benefits, works in synergy with maca root, a powerful adaptogen renowned for its ability to boost libido, enhance endurance, and balance hormones. This combination supports overall reproductive health and increases energy levels, making it beneficial for those looking to naturally enhance their sexual well-being.

Ingredients
- 2 tablespoons of cold-pressed castor oil
- 1 tablespoon of maca root powder
- 1 cup of warm almond milk
- 1 teaspoon of honey (optional, for sweetness)
- A pinch of cinnamon (optional, for flavor and blood circulation benefits)

Instructions
1. Warm the almond milk in a saucepan over low heat until it is just warm to the touch. Avoid boiling to preserve the nutrients.
2. Add the maca root powder to the warm almond milk and stir well to ensure it is fully dissolved.
3. Stir in the cold-pressed castor oil, mixing thoroughly to combine with the maca-infused almond milk.
4. If desired, add honey for sweetness and a pinch of cinnamon for enhanced flavor and additional circulatory benefits. Stir well.
5. Consume this libido-enhancing tonic once daily, preferably in the morning, to support sexual health and energy levels throughout the day.

Variations
- For a vegan-friendly version, ensure the honey is substituted with maple syrup or omitted according to personal preference.
- To enhance the tonic's energizing effects, add a teaspoon of raw cacao powder, which is also known for its ability to boost libido.

Storage tips

Prepare the Castor Oil and Maca Root Libido Enhancer fresh each time to ensure the maximum effectiveness of the ingredients. It is not recommended to store the prepared tonic as the active properties are best when consumed immediately after preparation.

Tips for allergens

If you have a nut allergy and cannot consume almond milk, substitute it with oat milk or coconut milk as a safe alternative. Always ensure that you are not allergic to maca root by performing a patch test or consulting with a healthcare provider before incorporating it into your routine.

Castor Oil and Shatavari Women's Wellness Drink

Beneficial effects

The Castor Oil and Shatavari Women's Wellness Drink is specifically formulated to support women's health, targeting hormonal balance, fertility, and overall vitality. Castor oil, with its rich nutritional profile, aids in detoxifying and stimulating the lymphatic system, while Shatavari, known as the "Queen of Herbs" in Ayurvedic medicine, is celebrated for its ability to support reproductive health, regulate menstrual cycles, and strengthen the female reproductive system. This wellness drink is an excellent choice for women seeking to enhance their health naturally.

Ingredients

- 2 tablespoons of cold-pressed castor oil
- 1 teaspoon of Shatavari powder
- 1 cup of warm almond milk
- Honey to taste (optional)

Instructions

1. Warm the almond milk in a saucepan over low heat until it is just warm to the touch. Avoid boiling to preserve the nutrients.
2. Stir in the Shatavari powder until it is completely dissolved in the warm almond milk.
3. Add the cold-pressed castor oil to the mixture and stir well to ensure all ingredients are fully combined.
4. If desired, sweeten the drink with honey to taste.
5. Consume this wellness drink in the morning on an empty stomach to maximize absorption and benefits.

Variations

- For added flavor and health benefits, include a pinch of cinnamon or cardamom to the drink. Both spices can enhance the taste and offer additional anti-inflammatory properties.
- If almond milk is not available, substitute with coconut milk or any plant-based milk of your choice for a similar creamy texture and nutritional profile.

Storage tips

It's best to prepare the Castor Oil and Shatavari Women's Wellness Drink fresh each time to ensure the potency of the ingredients. However, if you need to prepare it in advance, store the drink in the refrigerator for no more than 24 hours in a sealed glass container. Shake well before consuming.

Tips for allergens

If you are allergic to almonds, opt for a different plant-based milk to avoid any allergic reactions. For those sensitive to honey, it can be omitted or replaced with maple syrup as a natural sweetener. Always consult with a healthcare provider before incorporating new supplements into your diet, especially if you have specific health conditions or concerns.

Chapter 6: Practical Applications and Safety

Incorporating castor oil into daily routines offers a myriad of health and beauty benefits, yet understanding the practical applications and ensuring safety is paramount. Castor oil, revered for its healing properties, can be a powerful natural remedy when used correctly. However, to harness these benefits effectively, one must adhere to guidelines that ensure both safety and optimal results.

When integrating castor oil into health and beauty regimens, the choice of oil is crucial. Opting for cold-pressed, organic, and hexane-free castor oil ensures purity and potency, minimizing the risk of skin irritations or adverse reactions.

For topical applications, such as treating acne, promoting hair growth, or alleviating joint pain, understanding the correct method of application is essential. A patch test is recommended before widespread use to rule out allergic reactions. Applying a small amount of castor oil to a discreet skin area and waiting for 24 hours can help ensure compatibility. For hair treatments, massaging the oil into the scalp and through the hair can provide nourishment and enhance hair health, but it should be done sparingly to avoid excessive oiliness.

Regarding the use of castor oil packs, it is important to limit each session to 45-60 minutes and to not overuse, as excessive application can lead to adverse effects.

Safety considerations are paramount when using castor oil, especially for internal use. Although castor oil has been used as a natural laxative, internal consumption should be approached with caution. Only a small dosage, typically one teaspoon on an empty stomach, is recommended, and it should not be used as a long-term solution for constipation without consulting a healthcare provider. Pregnant and breastfeeding women should avoid internal use of castor oil due to its potential to induce labor.

Understanding the dosages and potential side effects is crucial for safe and effective use. Overuse of castor oil, whether topically or internally, can lead to side effects such as diarrhea, abdominal cramps, or skin irritation. It is also important to store castor oil properly, in a cool, dark place, to maintain its efficacy and prevent rancidity.

In summary, castor oil offers a versatile and potent natural remedy for a wide range of health and beauty concerns. By choosing the right type of oil, understanding the correct methods of application, and adhering to safety guidelines, individuals can safely incorporate castor oil into their wellness routines. Whether seeking to improve skin and hair health, support digestive function, or relieve pain and inflammation, castor oil, when used responsibly, can be a valuable addition to a holistic health regimen.

Incorporating Castor Oil into Daily Routine

Incorporating castor oil into your daily routine can be a transformative step towards enhancing your health and beauty regimen with a natural, versatile remedy. With its rich history and scientifically backed benefits, castor oil offers a holistic approach to wellness that aligns with the desires of those seeking chemical-free solutions. To seamlessly integrate castor oil into everyday life, consider the following practical applications tailored to address common health and beauty concerns.

Morning Rituals:
1. Start your day with a detoxifying castor oil pack. Apply it to your abdomen to support digestive health and stimulate lymphatic circulation. Ensure the pack is warm but not uncomfortably hot, and limit the application to 30 minutes to invigorate your body without overwhelming it.
2. Incorporate a few drops of castor oil into your skincare routine. Mix it with your favorite moisturizer to hydrate and heal dry skin, or apply it directly to acne-prone areas to leverage its antimicrobial properties.
3. Boost hair health by massaging a small amount of castor oil into the scalp and hair ends. This can stimulate growth, improve scalp health, and add a natural shine to your hair. For convenience, consider doing this every other day or incorporating it into your weekly hair care routine.

Evening Rituals:
1. Create a calming bedtime routine with a castor oil pack. Placing it on the liver area can aid in detoxification and promote relaxation before sleep. Remember to keep the application gentle, focusing on relaxation rather than intensive treatment.
2. Use castor oil as a natural makeup remover. Its thick viscosity is effective at dissolving makeup, dirt, and impurities, leaving the skin clean and moisturized. Follow up with your regular cleanser for a thorough clean.
3. Prepare a castor oil bath blend for a soothing, anti-inflammatory soak. Add a few tablespoons of castor oil to warm bath water, along with essential oils like lavender or chamomile, to relax muscles and moisturize the skin.

By incorporating castor oil into your daily health and beauty routines, you can harness its numerous benefits in a practical, enjoyable way. Remember to listen to your body's responses and adjust your use of castor oil accordingly, ensuring a safe and beneficial experience.

Safety, Dosages, and Side Effects

Navigating the world of natural remedies, especially castor oil, requires a balance between enthusiasm for its benefits and caution regarding its use. Castor oil, celebrated for its healing properties, can indeed be a potent ally in your health and beauty regimen when used with an understanding of its appropriate dosages and potential side effects. This knowledge not only ensures your safety but also maximizes the efficacy of castor oil in your wellness journey.

When considering the incorporation of castor oil into your routine, it's imperative to start with the premise that more is not always better. The effectiveness of castor oil does not linearly increase with its amount;

rather, there's an optimal threshold beyond which the benefits plateau or even reverse into undesirable effects. For topical applications, a few drops to a teaspoonful is generally sufficient, depending on the area of application. For internal use, particularly as a laxative, starting with a small dose, such as half a teaspoon on an empty stomach, is advisable. This amount can be adjusted based on individual tolerance and response, but it's crucial to not exceed two teaspoons in a single dose.

The potential side effects of castor oil, especially when taken orally, include diarrhea, abdominal cramps, nausea, and electrolyte imbalance with prolonged use. These effects stem from castor oil's powerful laxative properties, which, while beneficial in moderation, can lead to dehydration and nutrient depletion if overused. Pregnant women should avoid taking castor oil internally as it can induce labor, a property that has been both a traditional use and a cautionary note in medical circles.

In summary, the judicious use of castor oil, guided by an understanding of its dosages and potential side effects, is key to harnessing its benefits while minimizing risks. By starting with low doses, observing your body's reactions, and adjusting accordingly, you can safely incorporate castor oil into your wellness practices. Remember, the goal is to support your health and well-being, a journey that thrives on balance, patience, and informed choices. Whether you're using castor oil for its health benefits or its beauty enhancements, a respectful approach to its potency will ensure you reap the rewards it has to offer.

Chapter 7: Final Thoughts and Encouragement

Embarking on a journey with castor oil is akin to rediscovering a path to natural wellness that has been trodden by generations before us. The versatility and efficacy of castor oil, as detailed throughout this guide, offer a beacon of hope for those seeking to enhance their health and beauty through nature's bounty. The myriad recipes and applications presented serve not just as a testament to the oil's potency but as a toolkit for anyone ready to integrate these ancient practices into modern life.

As you stand at this juncture, equipped with knowledge and inspired by the possibilities that castor oil presents, remember that the journey to wellness is personal and unique. It's about finding balance, listening to your body, and making informed choices that resonate with your individual health and beauty goals. The steps laid out in this book are designed to empower you, offering guidance while encouraging personal experimentation and adaptation to fit your needs.

Let the stories of transformation and the scientific evidence bolster your confidence in the power of castor oil. Yet, approach each application with mindfulness, recognizing the importance of patience and consistency in witnessing tangible results. Your wellness journey with castor oil is not a quick fix but a commitment to nurturing your body and soul with nature's healing touch.

In moments of doubt or when results seem slow to manifest, lean on the community of fellow castor oil enthusiasts. Share experiences, seek advice, and draw encouragement from the collective wisdom and support that surrounds this ancient remedy.

As you move forward, let the principles of natural wellness guide your path. Embrace the journey with an open heart and mind, allowing the transformative power of castor oil to unfold in its own time. Your commitment to this natural elixir is not just a step towards achieving specific health and beauty goals but a deeper connection to the timeless wisdom of holistic healing.

Appendix

Glossary of terms

Understanding the terminology associated with castor oil is essential for harnessing its full potential in your health and beauty routines. Here are key terms defined to enrich your knowledge and application of castor oil:

- **Castor Oil**: Extracted from the seeds of the Ricinus communis plant, this vegetable oil is celebrated for its therapeutic properties.

- **Cold-Pressed**: This extraction method involves mechanically pressing the seeds without external heat, ensuring the oil retains its natural nutrients and therapeutic qualities.

- **Organic**: Castor oil labeled as organic is derived from plants grown without the use of synthetic pesticides, fertilizers, or genetically modified organisms, offering a pure and eco-friendly option.

- **Hexane-Free**: Indicates the absence of hexane, a chemical solvent, in the extraction process of castor oil, making it safer and more beneficial for health and environmental reasons.

- **Ricinoleic Acid**: A unique fatty acid found abundantly in castor oil, known for its anti-inflammatory, antibacterial, and analgesic (pain-relieving) properties, contributing to the oil's versatile uses.

- **Castor Oil Pack**: A compress made by soaking a piece of cloth in castor oil and placing it on the skin to support health through improved circulation and healing properties.

- **Laxative**: Castor oil acts as a stimulant laxative, encouraging bowel movements by increasing the movement of the intestines, often used to relieve temporary constipation.

- **Topical Application**: The direct application of a substance, in this case, castor oil, onto the skin for localized treatment or cosmetic purposes.

- **Internal Use**: Consuming a substance orally for medicinal benefits. Castor oil, when ingested in small quantities, can act as a laxative or support immune function.

- **Detoxification**: The process of removing toxins from the body. Castor oil is believed to support detoxification through its effects on the lymphatic system.

- **Lymphatic System**: A crucial part of the immune system, consisting of organs, lymph nodes, ducts, and vessels that transport lymph, a fluid containing white blood cells, throughout the body.

- **Antimicrobial**: Substances that kill or inhibit the growth of microorganisms, including bacteria and fungi. Castor oil's antimicrobial properties make it useful for treating skin infections and preserving cosmetic formulations.

- **Anti-inflammatory**: Refers to the property of a substance to reduce inflammation or swelling. Castor oil is widely used for its anti-inflammatory effects in various therapeutic applications.

- **Analgesic**: A type of medication that relieves pain. Castor oil's analgesic properties are beneficial for alleviating discomfort from ailments like arthritis and menstrual cramps.

- **Patch Test**: A method to test for allergic reactions by applying a small amount of a substance to the skin and observing for any signs of irritation or allergy, recommended before using new skincare products, including castor oil, extensively.

Thank you for embarking on this journey to natural health and beauty with the 'Castor Oil Bible' book. To express my gratitude for your choice, I'm delighted to offer you an **EXCLUSIVE BONUS**.

<u>Unlock the ultimate reading experience</u> with this exclusive **bonus**!

Simply **scan the QR code** and claim your reward today:

- **BONUS** - NATURAL CREATIONS: DIY BATH, BODY, and HERBAL ESSENTIALS – Ebook

SCAN ME

Small request:

Our work is done with great passion and commitment to produce a book that can meet ourreader's expectations.

If you liked this book and you would like to review it on Amazon, you will help us improve our products quality and help others in their journey towards complete self-sufficiency.

To do this is very simple: find the book among your orders or search for it directly on Amazon, and at the bottom of the sales page, you will find a button (on the left) that says "write a customer review". That's done. Thank you very much.

Made in the USA
Las Vegas, NV
15 September 2024